Emergency Psychiatry

Review of Psychiatry Series

John M. Oldham, M.D., M.S.
Michelle B. Riba, M.D., M.S.
Series Editors

Emergency Psychiatry

EDITED BY

Michael H. Allen, M.D.

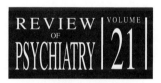

No. 3

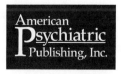

Washington, DC
London, England

Copyright © 2002 American Psychiatric Publishing, Inc.

07 06 05 04 03 02   7 6 5 4 3 2 1

ALL RIGHTS RESERVED

Manufactured in the United States of America on acid-free paper

American Psychiatric Publishing, Inc.
1400 K Street, N.W.
Washington, DC 20005
www.appi.org

The correct citation for this book is

Allen MH (editor): *Emergency Psychiatry* (Review of Psychiatry Series, Volume 21, Number 3; Oldham JM and Riba MB, series editors). Washington, DC, American Psychiatric Publishing, 2002

Library of Congress Cataloging-in-Publication Data
Emergency psychiatry / edited by Michael H. Allen.
     p. ; cm. — (Review of psychiatry ; v. 21, no. 3)
    Includes bibliographical references and index.
    ISBN 1-58562-070-X (alk. paper)
    1. Psychiatry. 2. Psychiatry—Miscellanea. 3. Mental health. 4. Hospitals—Emergency service. I. Allen, Michael H. II. Review of psychiatry series ; v. 21, 3.
    RC454.4 .E48 2002
    616.89′025—dc21

                                              2002022571

British Library Cataloguing in Publication Data
A CIP record is available from the British Library.

Contents

Chapter 3
Assessment and Treatment of Suicidal
Patients in an Emergency Setting   75

Peter L. Forster, M.D.
Linda H. Wu, B.A.

Chapter 4
Emergency Treatment of Agitation and
Aggression   115

J. P. Lindenmayer, M.D.
Martha Crowner, M.D.
Victoria Cosgrove, B.A.

Chapter 5

Psychosocial Interventions in the Psychiatric Emergency Service: A Skills Approach   **151**
Ronald C. Rosenberg, M.D.
Kerry J. Sulkowicz, M.D.

Contributors

Michael H. Allen, M.D.
Director of Inpatient Psychiatry, Colorado Psychiatric Health; Assistant Professor of Psychiatry, University of Colorado School of Medicine, Denver, Colorado

Richard E. Breslow, M.D.
Director of Crisis Services, Capital District Psychiatric Center; Clinical Associate Professor of Psychiatry, Albany Medical College, Albany, New York

Marc L. Copersino, Ph.D.
Postdoctoral Fellow, Department of Psychiatry, Johns Hopkins School of Medicine, Baltimore, Maryland

Victoria Cosgrove, B.A.
Research Scientist, Psychopharmacology Research Unit, Manhattan Psychiatric Center–Nathan Kline Institute for Psychiatric Research, New York, New York

Martha Crowner, M.D.
Clinical Associate Professor of Medicine, Department of Psychiatry, New York University School of Medicine; Attending Psychiatrist, Manhattan Psychiatric Center, New York, New York

Glenn W. Currier, M.D., M.P.H.
Director, Comprehensive Psychiatric Emergency Services, University of Rochester Medical Center; Assistant Professor of Psychiatry and Emergency Medicine, University of Rochester School of Medicine, Rochester, New York

Peter L. Forster, M.D.
Associate Clinical Professor of Psychiatry, University of California, San Francisco; Director, Gateway Psychiatric Services, San Francisco, California

John M. Oldham, M.D., M.S.
Dollard Professor and Acting Chairman, Department of Psychiatry, Columbia University College of Physicians and Surgeons, New York, New York

Michelle B. Riba, M.D., M.S.
Associate Chair for Education and Academic Affairs, Department of Psychiatry, University of Michigan Medical School, Ann Arbor, Michigan

Kerry J. Sulkowicz, M.D.
Clinical Associate Professor of Psychiatry and Faculty, New York University Psychoanalytic Institute, New York University Medical Center; President, The Boswell Group, New York, New York

J. P. Lindenmayer, M.D.
Clinical Professor, Department of Psychiatry, New York University School of Medicine; Director, Psychopharmacology Research Unit, Manhattan Psychiatric Center–Nathan Kline Institute for Psychiatric Research, New York, New York

Ronald C. Rosenberg, M.D.
Associate Director, Inpatient Psychiatric Services, North Shore University Hospital, Manhasset, New York

Mark R. Serper, Ph.D.
Associate Professor of Psychology, Hofstra University, Hempstead, New York; Assistant Professor of Psychiatry, New York University School of Medicine, New York, New York

Adam J. Trenton, B.A.
Research Assistant, Department of Psychiatry, University of Rochester School of Medicine, Rochester, New York

Linda H. Wu, B.A.
Research Associate, Gateway Psychiatric Services, San Francisco, California

Introduction to the Review of Psychiatry Series

John M. Oldham, M.D., M.S.
Michelle B. Riba, M.D., M.S., Series Editors

2002 REVIEW OF PSYCHIATRY SERIES TITLES

- *Cutting-Edge Medicine: What Psychiatrists Need to Know*
  EDITED BY NADA L. STOTLAND, M.D., M.P.H.
- *The Many Faces of Depression in Children and Adolescents*
  EDITED BY DAVID SHAFFER, F.R.C.P.(LOND), F.R.C.PSYCH.(LOND),
  AND BRUCE D. WASLICK, M.D.
- *Emergency Psychiatry*
  EDITED BY MICHAEL H. ALLEN, M.D.
- *Mental Health Issues in Lesbian, Gay, Bisexual, and Transgender Communities*
  EDITED BY BILLY E. JONES, M.D., M.S., AND MARJORIE J. HILL, PH.D.

There is a growing literature describing the stress–vulnerability model of illness, a model applicable to many, if not most, psychiatric disorders and to physical illness as well. Vulnerability comes in a number of forms. Genetic predisposition to specific conditions may arise as a result of spontaneous mutations, or it may be transmitted intergenerationally in family pedigrees. Secondary types of vulnerability may involve susceptibility to disease caused by the weakened resistance that accompanies malnutrition, immunocompromised states, and other conditions. In most of these models of illness, vulnerability consists of a necessary but not sufficient precondition; if specific stresses are avoided, or if they are encountered but offset by adequate protective factors, the disease does not manifest itself and the vulnerability may never be recognized. Conversely, there is increasing recognition of the role of stress as a precipitant of frank illness in vulnerable individuals and of the complex and subtle interactions among the environment, emotions, and neurodevelopmental, metabolic, and physiological processes.

In this country, the years 2001 and 2002 contained stress of unprecedented proportions, with the terrorist attacks on September 11 and the events that followed that terrible day. Although the contents of Volume 21 of the Review of Psychiatry were well established by that date and much of the text had already been written, we could not introduce this volume without thinking about the relevance of this unanticipated, widespread stress to the topics already planned.

Certainly, major depression is one of the prime candidates among the disorders in vulnerable populations that can be precipitated by stress. The information presented in *The Many Faces of Depression in Children and Adolescents*, edited by David Shaffer and Bruce D. Waslick, is, then, timely indeed. Already identified as a growing problem in youth—all too often accompanied by suicidal behavior—depression in children and adolescents is especially important to identify as early as possible. School-based screening services need to be widespread in order to facilitate both prevention of the disorder in those at risk and referral for effective treatment for those already experiencing symptomatic depression. Both psychotherapy and pharmacotherapy are well established as effective treatments for this condition, making recognition of its presence even more important. In New York alone, thousands of children lost at least one parent in the World Trade Center disaster, a catastrophic event precipitating not just grief but also major depression in the children and adolescents at risk.

We now know that stress, and depression itself, affect not just the brain but the body as well. New information about this brain–body axis is provided in *Cutting-Edge Medicine: What Psychiatrists Need to Know*, edited by Nada L. Stotland. Depression as an independent risk factor for cardiac death is one of the new findings reviewed in the chapter on the mind and the heart, as we understand more about the interactions among emotions, behavior, and cardiovascular functioning. Similarly, stress and mood are primary players in the homeostasis, or lack of it, of other body systems, such as the menstrual cycle and gastrointestinal functioning, also reviewed in this book. Finally, the massive increase in organ transplantation, in which medical advances have made it possible to neutralize the body's own immune responses against foreign tissue, represents a new frontier in which emotional stability is critical in donor and recipient.

Increasingly, medicine's front door is the hospital emergency service. Not just a place where triage occurs, though that remains an important and challenging function, the psychiatric emergency service needs to have expert clinicians who can perform careful assessments and initiate treatment. The latest thinking by psychiatrists experienced in emergency work is presented in *Emergency Psychiatry*, edited by Michael H. Allen. Certainly, psychiatric emergency services serve as one of the most critical components of the response network that needs to be in place to deal with a disaster such as the September 2001 attack and the bioterrorism events that followed.

Perhaps less obviously linked to those September events, *Mental Health Issues in Lesbian, Gay, Bisexual, and Transgender Communities*, edited by Billy E. Jones and Marjorie J. Hill, which reviews current thinking about gay, lesbian, bisexual, and transgender issues, reflects our changing world in other ways. A continuing process is necessary as we rethink our assumptions and challenge and question any prejudice or bias that may have infiltrated our thinking or may have been embedded in our traditional concepts. In this book, traditional notions are contrasted with newer thinking about gender role and sexual orientation, considering these issues from youth to old age, as we continue to try to differentiate the wide range of human diversity from what we classify as illness.

We believe that the topics covered in Volume 21 are timely and represent a selection of important updates for the practicing clinician. Next year, this tradition will continue, with books on trauma and disaster response and management, edited by Robert J. Ursano and Ann E. Norwood; on molecular neurobiology for the clinician, edited by Dennis S. Charney; on geriatric psychiatry, edited by Alan M. Mellow; and on standardized assessment for the clinician, edited by Michael B. First.

Preface

Michael H. Allen, M.D.

This book in the Review of Psychiatry series will attempt to meet two needs. Psychiatric emergencies are unpredictable and potentially catastrophic. Consequently mental health practitioners of all types in all settings must be prepared for crises like suicidal ideation, agitation and aggression, and acute confusion.

For various reasons, such crises are becoming more common. Substance abuse has increased, while access to both inpatient and outpatient mental health and substance abuse services has declined. This has been associated with a rise in emergency room visits for these problems. Many of these episodes will be unreimbursed, which discourages facilities from organizing services of this type. This forces larger numbers of patients to rely on the few services that are available and often to move constantly among mandated providers because of lack of regular and effective care in the community.

Two things happen then. Many providers of more routine care find themselves dealing with increasingly urgent and complex problems in settings that are not intended for that purpose. Patients with substance abuse, confusion, agitation, and self-aggressive behavior must now be managed in community settings. To the degree that serious problems result in hospitalization at all, the hospitalization is brief and the underlying problem is attenuated but not resolved. Consequently, many clinicians feel pressure to keep their emergency assessment and management skills honed.

On the other hand, in some places the volume of emergencies is such that it becomes necessary to organize around them. Hence, in recent years, specialized services have emerged that have begun to evolve as did emergency medicine in the direction of intensivism. Intensivists in mental health, as in emergency medicine, must have expertise in assessing critical problems, differentiating urgent and emergent from nonurgent, providing stabilizing or initial definitive treatment, and transfering to the appropriate level of care. They also must be able to provide basic assessment for all mental health problems for those who lack access to other care settings.

Surprisingly, no formal training in emergency mental health was required, even for psychiatrists, until rather recently. Most psychiatry training programs had emergency room service obligations, but indirect supervision was the rule. Only since 1994 have psychiatric residency programs been required to provide an organized emergency psychiatry experience in addition to call. This has been a challenge for some programs because of the lack of an appropriately supervised setting. For other kinds of mental health professionals, preparation for psychiatric emergencies has been even less methodical. Some psychiatric emergencies appear in the core competencies for emergency physicians but not the Accreditation Council on Graduate Medical Education program requirements.

This book then attempts to meet the needs of both the generalist, who must be prepared for eventualities that are rare in most settings but life threatening in some cases, and the intensivist, for whom these situations are common and require some standardization. All of the contributions here reflect a belief that emergency patients deserve the same thoughtful, quality care to which they are entitled under any other circumstances, regardless of the time of day or place of occurrence.

First, it is helpful to understand the nature of psychiatric emergencies and the settings that have evolved to manage them. These include observation units, mobile teams, and crisis residences as well as the traditional emergency room. Richard Breslow, in Chapter 1, provides an overview of this topic.

Given the wide variation in complexity and volume of mental health crises and the resources available, schemas for emergency assessment and resource allocation are important. Glenn Currier and colleagues provide, in Chapter 2, a review of medical, psychiatric, substance use, and cognitive assessment and describe efficient approaches to triage, "medical clearance," and psychiatric assessment.

Actual or incipient violence, directed at self or others, accounts for or complicates a large fraction of psychiatric emergencies. The Surgeon General recently made suicide prevention a health priority, and a great deal of attention has been focused on this problem. Peter Forster and Linda Wu, in their chapter on the assessment of the suicidal patient, review the modifiable and unmodifiable factors associated with suicide risk and offer an evidence-based approach to the evaluation and management of the suicidal patient.

Agitation and aggression have recently become more topical because of efforts to decrease utilization of physical and so-called chemical restraint. Agitation is an ephemeral state occurring in a wide variety of conditions, and it has been poorly studied. Aggression occurs frequently in this state, but most aggression is unrelated to psychiatric status. J. P. Lindenmayer and colleagues review this complex area of neurobiology, characterize the assessment of patients with aggression or agitation, and illuminate the basis for clinical management of dangerous patients.

Last, but not least, is the care in emergency mental health care. Therapeutic approaches to the patient in crisis have been neglected for many years, but Ronald Rosenberg and Kerry Sulkowicz, in their chapter on psychosocial intervention, attempt to describe how various psychotherapeutic theories and skills developed for office settings may be adapted to understanding and aiding individuals in the compressed time frame of the emergency. The central premise of Rosenberg's work is that skillful use of the emergency interview can not only facilitate the emergency assessment but also promote incremental change and influence attitudes toward continued treatment.

Chapter 1

Structure and Function of Psychiatric Emergency Services

Richard E. Breslow, M.D.

Psychiatric Emergency Services and Psychiatric Emergencies

Psychiatric emergency services (PESs) are designed to respond to psychiatric emergencies as they arise (Gerson and Bassuk 1980). Psychiatric emergencies are acute situations of sufficient gravity to warrant immediate assessment and treatment. An *emergency* is a set of circumstances in which a catastrophic outcome is thought to be imminent and the resources available to understand and deal with the situation are unavailable at the time and place of the occurrence. Emergencies often materialize suddenly despite prolonged gestation. An emergency may occur at any time. The absence of resources adequate to deal with a situation may provoke an emergency or contribute to the sense of urgency. Any marked change in a person's mental status that activates a response in the support system to seek help may come under the responsibility of the emergency psychiatric system (Munizza et al. 1993). When emergencies are detected, there is a response by the person, support system, therapist, clinic, family doctor, police, mobile team, emergency room, insurance company, or managed care organization. These are the stakeholders in emergency psychiatric services because the response generally is referral for emergency psychiatric evaluation.

In psychiatry the common emergencies are suicide, acute

psychosis, other mental status change, substance abuse, and behavioral disturbance. Data collected by Dhossche (2000) indicate that 38% of psychiatric emergencies involve suicidal ideation or suicidal behavior. Breslow et al. (1996a) reported that 32% of patients presenting to a PES were acutely intoxicated with alcohol or other substances of abuse; 17% of the overall population who presented had a primary diagnosis of substance abuse or dependence. Wingerson et al. (2001) studied 2,419 consecutive patients who visited a crisis triage unit and found that 30% had unipolar depression, 26% psychosis, 20% substance use disorder, 14% bipolar disorder, 4% adjustment disorder, 3% anxiety disorder, and 2% dementia. Allen got diagnostic estimates from survey data in compiling his expert consensus guideline work on treatment of behavioral emergencies (Allen et al. 2001) and reported the following averages of the expert's survey answers: 23% unipolar depression, 28% psychosis, 25% substance use disorder, 13% bipolar, and 5% dementia (M. Allen, M.D., personal communication, October 2001).

Classification of Medical Emergencies and Applications to Psychiatry

Work has been done over the past quarter century in emergency medicine to define the nature of medical emergencies and classify the emergency systems that respond. The first guidelines used a "horizontal" system that went from level 1, with 24-hour emergency care with an emergency medicine specialist on site and immediate consultation capacity with specialists, to level 4, which implies availability of standby care and, when necessary, first aid and referral to a facility that can handle the problem (Commission on Emergency Medical Services 1971). Ten years later this system was supplemented with a "vertical" categorization that defines a facility's emergency care capability for specific critically ill patient groups, such as behavioral, trauma, burn, spinal cord, and cardiac patients (Commission on Emergency Medical Services 1982). Such a system allows more flexibility in allocation of resources, since every facility does not have to be level 1 for every potential patient care emergency. More recently, Schneider et al.

(1998) developed a position paper to clarify the role of emergency medicine as having the mission of evaluating, managing, treating, and preventing unexpected illness and injury. In 2001, a practice analysis was done to assist in developing a core content for the clinical practice of emergency medicine (Hockberger et al. 2001). The content shows how an emergency physician modifies the specific tasks necessary to perform appropriate patient care on the basis of a matrix of patient acuity, where *acuity* is defined as how urgently the patient needs care.

Psychiatry does not have a formal level system for delivery of services in psychiatric emergencies. However, it is possible to classify informal equivalents to the level system. Hospital emergency departments (EDs) have become the focus of health care in medical emergencies and for more general medical problems when there are problems in accessing other components of the health system (Bell et al. 1991). Factors such as lack of health insurance, poverty, limited education, membership of a vulnerable population, or limited hours of operation of health care facilities (Johnson and Thornicroft 1995) throw the burden of much general medical care on the ED. Since EDs were federally mandated by the Emergency Medical Treatment and Active Labor Act (EMTALA) to provide a medical screening examination and treatment for all patients who present themselves for care, the emergency service has become the only guaranteed access point to the health care system. Psychiatric patients are particularly prone to access problems such as those delineated above. Psychiatric emergencies are unpredictable and, for many hours of the day, low-volume occurrences. Therefore, it is frequently difficult to have resources available at the site of the problem. This has led to dependence on assets that are always available to the community, such as the ED. The equivalent of a level 3 or 4 medical emergency service is the use of the medical ED for the delivery of psychiatric services.

We may continue to try to fit psychiatric services in a rough and approximate fashion into this analogy to the classification scheme of medical emergencies. The model of the psychiatric consultant to the ED (the *consultation model*), which will be discussed in more depth later in this chapter, is the equivalent of a level 2 service. The *specialized psychiatric emergency service, or PES, model* in this analogy would be the equivalent of a level 1 service. This model will also be discussed in greater depth later in this chapter. Recent work from Canada has described a model of an *integrated psychiatric emergency service* (Kates et al. 1996). This service has evolved from the integration of five separate, hospital-run emergency psychiatric services into a single service to render care to an entire medium-sized city. Psychiatric emergencies are handled centrally in one facility with a well-staffed emergency psychiatry team, and admissions then go to each of the participating hospitals. Perhaps this regional approach brings us in psychiatry closest to approximating the more sophisticated and differentiated "vertical" categorization of services that emergency medicine has developed.

As we try to assimilate some of these approaches to categorizing emergency services, it is helpful to try to articulate some of the goals for psychiatric emergency care to serve as a kind of measuring stick of how far we have come and what still needs to be accomplished.

Goals for Psychiatric Emergency Care

The first goal is *timely rendering of psychiatric emergency care.* As already discussed, emergencies frequently involve a mismatch of needs and resources, and quickly addressing the mismatch can significantly ameliorate the problem. Waiting times in EDs can often be quite extensive. This is exacerbated for patients with psychiatric problems, particularly when there are a number of patients in acute medical crisis utilizing the service. A separate PES can be helpful in this regard, but since staffing is much more limited than at the ED, when a number of patients arrive at the same time, it takes a long time to be seen. Appropriate mental health specialists should be available. A mixture of mental health disciplines operating as a team is desirable, given that patients present with a variety of medical, psychiatric, and social problems.

The second goal is *access to care*—that is, to have care that is local and community based. It is undesirable to have patients in the midst of an acute psychiatric emergency travel long distances for immediate stabilization. Sometimes it is necessary after the stabilization to use facilities at greater distances to obtain more definitive care. Over a century ago, Jarvis described the "distance decay" phenomenon—that greater use of psychiatric services is positively correlated with nearness to the psychiatric hospital (Jarvis 1851). "County drift," the tendency of chronic psychiatric patients to move from outlying counties to the central county containing the psychiatric hospital, may partially account for some of Jarvis's effect (Breslow et al. 1998). This research indicates that the more services are provided locally, the less this "drift" occurs, preventing the facilities in the central county from getting swamped. Some in the emergency psychiatry community have suggested fostering the opposite trend of organizing the more comprehensive PES by region, since such facilities are too expensive to be maintained in every locality (Allen 1999; Rae 1997). Obviously, some balance must be struck between the provision of some select specific services at the local level and the broader coverage of the comprehensive PES.

The third goal is *safety/stabilization and assessment*. The importance of a good assessment of the situation to accomplishing this goal cannot be overstated. In the case of the suicidal patient, determination must be made as soon as possible of what will keep the patient safe. In the patient with acute psychosis or mental status changes, the role of masquerading medical conditions and medical comorbidities should be considered and treated (Buckley 1994). Substance abuse is a frequent accompaniment of psychiatric emergencies and should always be part of the differential diagnosis, since there is a well-documented tendency to leave it out (Elangovan et al. 1993; Szuster et al. 1990). Behavioral disturbance and, more particularly, agitation have a high likelihood of attracting significant community attention. Before an intervention with medication is made, it is most important to determine whether there is a causal medical etiology or substance abuse issue that should be managed first. Noncoercive techniques—verbal intervention; "cooling off"; offering food, beverage, or smoke; assistance; problem solving—can help the situation markedly. Medication offered as part of a "plan of care," not chemical restraint, is the standard (Allen et al. 2001).

The fourth goal is *continuity of care*—that is, to respect the patient by offering continuity of care that is rendered at the least restrictive level possible. Continuity may be difficult to achieve, because, almost by definition, an emergency service is outside of the usual systems of care. PES visits are most likely to occur during hours when psychiatric resources in the community are closed. This highlights the value of the more comprehensive services, since they frequently have extensive arrangements for exchange of information and services with community-based providers. Mobile teams and admission diversion programs are frequently based in the PES. The PES may have an extended evaluation capacity that permits more time for stabilization of the patient and waiting until resources are available to treat the patient at less restrictive levels than that represented by inpatient hospitalization. The goal of treatment at the least restrictive level could even lead to the use of some of these programs to enable handling of the psychiatric emergency without the direct use of the PES itself. Crisis hospitalization, mobile teams, crisis residences, and managed care have all evolved in just this fashion to meet these needs.

Models for Delivery of Services in Psychiatric Emergencies

Consultation

The general model for delivery of psychiatric services in a medical emergency room is the consultant relationship. The patient is first seen by the medical doctors in the ED. After assessment and treatment are rendered, the psychiatric consultant is called to respond and evaluate. If the patient is to be admitted medically, this evaluation may be centered around management recommendations to the medical staff. Sometimes arrangements need to be made for ongoing psychiatric care and special observation on the medical unit. If the patient is medically "cleared," the consultation frequently revolves around transactions related to the need for psychiatric admission or outpatient referral. In either case, the psychiatrist, who usually has general coverage duties elsewhere, comes to the emergency department to see the patient, make an assessment, propose treatment, and recommend a disposition (Stebbins and Hardman 1993).

This model has the advantage of flexible use of physician time. Physicians can cover many different services and may be based on the inpatient unit or the outpatient clinic. In the after-hours situation, the physician can cover from home or private office. Nursing staff needs are minimized, since the ED staff are responsible for all care. A general medical evaluation is guaranteed for all patients. This feature is quite valuable, since mental status changes that generate ED visits frequently have organic causes. There should be good communication between medicine and psychiatry, since all parties to the consultation are physically located in the ED (McClelland 1983).

However, there are so many deficiencies to the consultation model that major modifications have been needed. The work of Gerson and Bassuk (1980) served a key role in organizing the thinking around what is necessary and desirable as an alternative to this model. The major modifications that have been needed have sometimes been accomplished with the help of legislative intervention, as in the case of New York (Oldham et al. 1990) and New Jersey (Kane et al. 1993).

The physical plant can be one of the most troubling issues facing existing PESs because, in many cases, they begin as stretchers in the ED. This poses several problems for the host ED, mental health consultants, patients, and families. Hospitals must confront the issue of whether to devote space to a separate PES. The organization of space in the ED does not allow for the privacy and ability to separate conflicting parties that may be crucial to a proper assessment. Psychiatric patients tend to be regarded as a nuisance or sometimes even a hindrance to the work of the ED because they frequently have accompanying behavioral disturbance (Comstock 1983). It is difficult to take into account the needs of an irritable or overstimulated patient in a busy ED. The impulsive or paranoid patient who may try to elope can be a major impediment to the work of the ED. Agitated patients may require restraint or seclusion, and suicidal patients require special observation.

Staff of the ED frequently develop a negative mind-set toward those with psychiatric emergencies, with the assumption that these emergencies are more volitional and less "genuine" than a true medical emergency. The negative mind-set extends to family members as well, who cannot be handled adequately in the available space and may be viewed as obstacles to rapid disposition (Barton 1974) The negative mind-set may even include a negative attitude toward the psychiatric consultant; there is an implicit, or at times more overt, demand to "get your patient out of my emergency room." Given these constraints, time pressures become pervasive, with one study showing that the average evaluation was done in under 15 minutes (Baxter et al. 1968).

This issue of the time course of evaluations presents perhaps the most fundamental conflict between the medical and the psychiatric emergency (Breslow et al. 1997). In the medical emergency, the high-acuity patient is generally in a life-threatening situation and must be seen and treated as rapidly as possible and then transferred (Hu 1993; Saunders 1987). The high-acuity psychiatric emergency patient may need rapid attention to prevent self-harm or harm to others. Once this is accomplished, longer time periods can be very helpful in allowing the immediate crisis to pass, letting acute intoxication resolve, noting and tracking changes in mental status, getting additional history and records, making contact with family members, and reapproaching the patient after some calming down to better establish a therapeutic alliance.

In the consultation model, the psychiatrist is always pulled from other clinical services to see a patient in an emergency situation. The whole process is viewed as, at best, an inconvenience and, at worst, a significant disruption, rather than as an end in itself. In this model, emergency work is regarded as undesirable and relegated to the most junior staff. Frequently, staff in training, such as residents, are handling emergencies largely on their own with limited or no direct supervision and few learning opportunities.

Specialized Psychiatric Emergency Services

The problems with the consultation model described above served as a tremendous impetus for the development of more comprehensive PESs (Breslow et al. 1996c; Hughes 1993; Oldham and DeMasi 1995). These comprehensive services usually are hospital based in conjunction with a large medical center or university-based medical school and residency teaching program. Allen (1999) has cited his experience that services with 3,000 or more visits per year tend to have a separate PES. These services are major investments in space and staffing. They must have sufficient space to allow for privacy and confidentiality and enough calm and quiet to enable staff to conduct an evaluation. The separation in space has many beneficial aspects, such as improved ability to observe patients, adequate areas to use for patients requiring special observation, family areas, "quiet room," and areas to be used for seclusion and restraint if those behavioral interventions should be needed. The chance to separate behaviorally disturbed patients helps the operation of the ED and benefits these patients as well by providing a quieter area in which to calm down (Hankoff et al. 1974). This ensures less "scapegoating" of both psychiatric patients and staff. It also provides a better opportunity to pay attention to the needs of patient's families; their questions can be answered and their participation can be utilized to improve the treatment plan (Barton 1974). Most services have direct access to the outside for "walk-in patients" that is also capable of accommodating ambulances. Some services accomplish this by close proximity to the medical ED. This entrance frequently needs to have a special locking system to prevent patient elopements. The PES generally has a waiting area; an area for collection of triage information; a nursing station, including a locked medication room; a physical examination room; offices for conducting patient interviews; a staff work area, which usually has "status" boards that help to track what work needs to be done; a patient lounge; a staff lounge; offices for permanent staff; patient bedrooms; bathrooms and shower rooms with safety features for suicidal patients; a patient dining area; special observation and behavior management rooms, as delineated earlier; and space to house the mobile crisis team if the two services are combined or work in close coordination.

Patient and staff safety are major considerations in designing the physical space. Many patients require a high level of supervision, so a design that allows staff to observe the entire patient care area from a central location can be a desirable configuration. Interior windows that permit staff to see into interview rooms and bedrooms contribute to a sense of security for the staff. The privacy needs of patients must be balanced against the need for supervision. New security systems are based on video camera surveillance and personal alarms. Cameras are installed to view corridors, patient day areas, the smoking patio, and certain rooms. Split-screen monitors are placed in the staff work room and the nursing station to allow better observation of these areas. All staff carry personal alarms; if the alarm is set off, computer screens in the assessment area and the safety department flash a diagram of the PES with the area where the alarm was set off in red, and a picture of the staff person who set off the alarm is indicated on the screen.

A separate emergency facility also involves separate staffing. This enables recruitment of doctors, nurses, psychologists, and social workers with an interest in psychiatric emergencies who will be able to see these patients not as "nuisances" but as having illnesses requiring treatment (Blais and Georges 1969). This also allows staff to develop over time the specialized skills necessary to treat these patients. The group most interested in this area tend to be those most motivated to work in the PES. A "critical mass" of professional staff can accumulate more competence at rendering services in acute psychiatric emergencies than standard ED workers. In a similar fashion to the separate space requirements described above, these considerations of staffing also constitute a major investment. Around-the-clock coverage by psychiatrists is a crucial component of the PES model. One reason that physician direction of crisis services is so important is the frequency and severity of medical syndromes that mimic, complicate, or accompany mental illness. A high index of suspicion for organic conditions is necessary and the skills to identify them are essential in emergency settings. In addition to allowing screening for medical problems, psychiatrist participation helps to achieve more rapid diagnosis and initiation of psychiatric treatment.

The development of the PES model has been viewed as a major advance in correcting the deficiencies of the consultation model developed earlier (Hughes 1993). However, the PES model itself is not without its downside. The first rule is that it always requires more staff to cover a separate service than a combined service. Services separated from the ED need their own space, equipment, security systems, and specialized nursing, psychology, and social work staff. Full-time psychiatric coverage can also add a major operating expense. Sometimes the additional mental health "dollars" needed to fund the more comprehensive type of PES means fewer available dollars to fund other needed mental health programs such as psychiatric outreach, outpatient care, crisis residential services, or services for special populations such as children or the elderly.

Separation of the two services raises the possibility of less thorough medical evaluations as the medical staff of the ED hurry to get behaviorally disturbed patients out to the PES as soon as possible (Breslow et al. 1999). Patients who present first to the PES might not get the medical evaluation needed at all, unless psychiatric staff are attuned to the issue of possible underlying organic dysfunction. Communication might not be as good between medical and psychiatric staff when the services are separated. Patients, as well as their families, may feel stigmatized by being sent to a PES, rather than being treated in the ED. Sometimes they state that they do not want to be in a place with "crazy people." If they observe some disturbed behavior or locked doors, they may find the experience frightening.

Crisis Hospitalization

Crisis hospitalization has developed into a useful disposition alternative for the emergency service. In many instances it has enabled avoidance of longer-term standard psychiatric hospitalization while allowing for better treatment planning than immediate discharge from the PES. Many psychiatric emergencies are a function of a transient crisis confronted by patients with problems related to a personality disorder or substance abuse. These crises can be resolved with brief interventions, but the time frame may go considerably beyond what can be accommodated in the usual course of an emergency contact. Services have evolved along the lines of a 24-hour format that stresses the importance of making serial observations of the patient, maximizing the use of collaterals in the community, and actively engaging the treatment staff. Usually, a hospital-based setting is used for this purpose. This setting may have a formal or informal status within another medical or psychiatric service, or it may be organized as a unit associated with the PES. Involuntary and dangerous patients are acceptable, in contrast to the crisis residence (described later in this section), where patients must be cooperative.

Two models of crisis hospitalization have developed with different capabilities and goals (Breslow et al. 1995). The first provides extended observation or 23-hour bed availability. This model has been studied in several different contexts (Gillig et al. 1989; Ianzito et al. 1978; Kane et al. 1993). In many services, the focus is on the ability to hold the patient overnight when necessary to make community contacts in the morning. Potential additional benefits are in clarifying the reasons for the presentation and taking advantage of the rapid spontaneous resolution of many crises. "Filtering" of substance abuse emergencies is one example (Breslow et al. 1996a). Observation alone can potentially divert inappropriate admissions caused by misdiagnosis and limit the need for appropriate but predictably brief admissions.

The 72-hour bed model of crisis hospitalization was originally characterized by Weisman et al. (1969) and Rhine and Mayerson (1971). It was further developed by Comstock (1983) and Breslow et al. (1993). The concept was adopted as part of the New York State CPEP model and incorporated into formally licensed extended observation units (Oldham and DeMasi 1995; Oldham et al. 1990). Flexibility is provided if patients can actually be admitted to the PES for a few days. The same utilization review criteria that are used for standard inpatient admissions apply. Patients must have significant functional impairment or mental illness with threats to self or others sufficient to warrant inpatient treatment. A number of psychiatric beds (usually 2–12), sometimes called "holding beds," are designated for the purpose of these "very short hospitalization" units. It is usually best for these beds to have their own identity by being physically located on or near the PES.

The profile of those who could make positive use of this service would be those who require hospitalization for a condition that would be expected to improve in a brief time period. Personality disorder patients, who by definition have limited personality coping resources, frequently will develop suicidal ideation or gestures under stress. These patients respond dramatically to the short, focused nature of crisis hospitalization. They will strive to meet the expectations of the short stay and tend to regress much less than when they are hospitalized on a standard unit. Chronically mentally ill patients, if they are well connected with community treatment programs and are reacting to acute but transient stressors, may also respond favorably to crisis hospitalization. Patients who are abusing alcohol or other drugs but are no longer acutely intoxicated may still have substantial changes in mental status during the immediate postintoxication period. Crisis hospitalization makes possible a longer period in which to allow evaluation and resolution of these changes.

Community service providers such as case managers, supervised apartment programs, halfway houses, outpatient clinics, and continuing treatment programs view the possibility of crisis hospitalization as beneficial. The program maintains the morale of both the patient and his or her community supports. Community service providers and patients often see return to standard hospitalization as a failure. Crisis hospitalization allows both parties respite and time to mobilize defenses or to adjust treatment strategies to allow the patient to return to the community rapidly. We have found that patients already well connected with treatment in the community can be discharged much more readily (Breslow et al. 1995).

A group of emergency psychiatrists has developed specific techniques and advocated for definitive treatment in the PES (Forster and King 1994a, 1994b; Allen 1996). In the definitive treatment model, medications and psychotherapy are begun in the PES to shorten the total time needed to ameliorate the presenting problem. Initiation of antipsychotic and antianxiety medication in the emergency service has always been a useful practice, but use of antidepressants has been discouraged because of the concern about toxicity on overdose. Availability of newer antidepressants associated with much less toxicity has changed this (Freemantle et al. 1994; Kapur et al. 1992), and now emergency psychiatrists are using these agents (Brodsky and Pieczynski 1985; Glick 2000). A method for the rapid administration of divalproex sodium has been reported as safe and effective and is in use in some PES settings (Hirschfeld et al. 1999). This emphasis on initiation of treatment has led to interest in the use of atypical antipsychotic medications in the PES, since they have the potential for better compliance (Currier 2000).

Mobile Teams

Mobile systems of care have originated in an almost bewildering number of variations in localities throughout this country and in Europe to meet perceived community needs. The earliest systems developed over 25 years ago on the basis of an "activist" approach to the problems of mental illness and their relationship to social problems. One of the early units described reliance on a family system perspective as the model for care (Bengelsdorf and Alden 1987). The idea was to see the patient in the midst of the support system so as to intervene at an early stage and prevent further deterioration. Assessment and treatment could be directed toward the system itself to help resolve a family crisis, to connect patients with clinics or social service resources, or to advocate for the patient. The widespread belief was that such systems prevent inpatient psychiatric admission. It was thought that they could even eliminate the need for more traditional sources of emergency care, such as EDs and the PES (Granovetter 1975; Ruiz et al. 1973; West et al. 1980).

In contrast to these early hopes, there are few actual data demonstrating the effectiveness of mobile teams (Geller et al. 1995). A controlled study of localities with and without mobile teams failed to demonstrate an impact on admission rates to psychiatric hospitals (Fisher et al. 1990). Most of the other data collected on mobile teams are uncontrolled; counts are provided of the number of mobile contacts, and each is considered a prevention of hospitalization without consideration of base rates of hospitalization or the patient's status at longitudinal follow-up. These findings are of particular concern, since mobile services are not covered by most insurance plans, including Medicare, and are often publicly supported with taxpayer funds through county or state grants. This creates substantial pressure to justify these programs on the basis of cost effectiveness.

The challenge to investigate the effectiveness of mobile teams in a more rigorous fashion has begun to be met. One well-designed randomized study of community outreach versus hospital-based care did demonstrate greater symptom improvement, more patient satisfaction, and dramatically less use of inpatient psychiatric services among those assigned to the outreach care (Merson et al. 1992). Patients were randomized to a multidisciplinary community-based early intervention team or a conventional hospital-based psychiatric service with clinic facilities. The authors felt that the better outcome in the community group was from a greater ability to ensure follow-up with the outreach team, compared with the clinic, where many of the patients did not keep or receive continuing appointments. A program evaluation of the New York State CPEP program found that mobile crisis patients were more often referred by family, more often psychotic, and twice as likely to be severely ill and violent as were similar patients seen in the ED, but they were still less likely to be admitted to the hospital (Oldham and DeMasi 1995). Guo et al. (2001), using a quasi-experimental design with an ex post facto matched control group, found that community-based mobile crisis services resulted in a lower rate of hospitalization than did hospital-based interventions. The authors also described consumer characteristics associated with the risk of hospitalization.

It is possible to differentiate types of mobile crisis services with different rationales underlying the service. Gillig (1995) has described levels of mobile outreach. The first level deals with emergent circumstances and involves acute emergencies in the community, such as with suicidal, acutely psychotic, behaviorally disturbed, or threatening patients. Frequently, such outreach involves either a police emergency or a mobile team intervention to prevent a police emergency. In many instances, public demand for such services was originally created by some high-profile incident that occurred that created such publicity that local officials were able to justify expenditure of taxpayer funds to finance the service. This type of service does not function to prevent admission but, rather, works in the opposite sense of a "case finder" for the emergency service, since most of these patients are referred to the emergency service. Subsequently, the patients are held for stabilization and, in many cases, are admitted to the psychiatric inpatient unit. Mental health practitioners involved in this activity require special training and must interact with the police in a coordinated manner (Zealberg et al. 1992). Mobile outreach often develops as a means of extending mental health expertise to individuals and agencies, including the police, that are involved with the mentally ill in the community. Services may be closely allied with or even housed in the PES and are available on a 24-hour basis. Some problems can be resolved directly by the team in the community. If hospital services are deemed necessary, transportation to the hospital may be accomplished by experienced mental health professionals with less force and more dignity. A step down from the emergent type of mobile crisis services are the teams that deal with urgent situations of more moderate acuity. The team might not be available on a 24-hour basis, and response times may be 1 or 2 days rather than the immediate response of the emergent team. These teams rely on the police to handle imminently suicidal or homicidal patients. They focus more on outreach and "maintenance in the community" and less on "case finding." A further step down is to the mobile clinics that deal with still lower acuity situations in the community. One approach is to use the model of the "psychiatric house call" to deliver home treatment to patients (Chiu and Primeau 1991; Soreff 1983; Tufnell et al. 1985). Home treatment is beneficial in engaging reluctant patients, strengthening the support network, working with the entire environment, collaborating with the family in therapy, dealing with the social service system, and providing medication for patients who do not respond to hospitalization. This mobile approach has even been adapted for outreach to homeless persons through the use of vans and good communication equipment to provide the benefits of the home visit approach (Cohen et al. 1984). The multidisciplinary team approach has been the prevailing model, with a psychiatrist, a psychiatric nurse, and a social worker constituting the mobile unit. Units are available only when the mobile team members are working. Referrals come from phone calls to the mobile unit made by family members, neighbors, clergymen, and assorted others.

Mobile services to lower-acuity patients can be organized using the model of an *outreach team*. These teams are suitable for rendering care to those who do not keep traditional clinic appointments or even use ED services. The team can help maintain the patient in the community and provide care for less well served populations such as the homeless, the elderly, and mentally ill substance abusers (Gillig et al. 1990). This type of outreach lends itself as well to aftercare services for patients who are readmitted repeatedly because they discontinue their medication and relapse (Rubinstein 1972). Another variant of this approach is the *admission diversion team*, which strives to provide psychotherapy, interim medication, and support to connect the patient to clinic care, social service, and housing options. The team intervention may begin at the PES with patients who do not need to be admitted but who have many acute psychiatric and social service needs. The team intervention is designed to be time limited, with treatment continuing in more standard outpatient settings. When housing is an issue, some teams assist in shelter placement and follow-up with regular shelter rounds to track the patients and provide supportive services. Emergency case management and provision for transportation to and from services can be part of the overall team responsibility. The variety of different types of mobile teams undoubtedly allows a wider and more diverse population to be served by the emergency mental health system.

Crisis Residences

Crisis residential treatment has become another component of emergency psychiatric care in many localities (Goodwin and Lyons 2001; Lamb and Lamb 1984; Mosher and Menn 1982; Stroul 1988). There is no ideal model for such a program, since one critical element of a successful crisis residence is its ability to adapt and to assume many forms, depending on the needs of a particular community and the local patterns of use of emergency services. The intention is to provide diversion from the emergency service to an acute care residential setting, rather than to use psychiatric hospitalization. Many services function on direct referral from the PES, but others can be accessed directly by the mobile team or various case managers, by-passing the need for a PES visit. Patients are referred to a specially prepared residential setting that may consist of a foster home setting for up to 2 individuals or a larger group home model of 6–15 clients.

In the *family-based crisis home,* carefully selected and trained families provide short-term housing/support to persons in acute psychiatric crisis. Professional staff support the family sponsors with case management services, nursing, and psychiatric backup to adjust medication, maintain compliance, and provide emergency hospitalization if needed. The advantage is in providing a less restrictive, less stigmatizing, less traumatic, more normative environment for the patient to resolve the psychiatric crisis. The economic benefit of avoiding hospitalization and perhaps shortening the duration of treatment may be considerable.

The *group home* model (Fields and Weisman 1995) adds the elements of therapeutic milieu, group support and feedback, and staffing by paraprofessionals who bring valuable community experience and different perspectives to the intervention. Some staff members may themselves have been consumers of mental health services and can draw on these experiences to relate better to the patients in crisis. These factors can be powerful tools in helping to bring about resolution of the psychiatric emergency. The emphasis is on a problem-solving approach and the need to work on a task in cooperation with others to get the patient to focus more quickly, avoiding the regression that institutionalization fosters. Programs may exclude the most severe emergencies, such as those involving acutely suicidal or violent patients or patients with medical problems. The usual time frame for resolution of the emergency is up to 2 weeks, when the expectation is for discharge to another level of care.

Managed Care

The relationship of managed care to PESs is complex. On the one hand, managed care borrows heavily from the emergency psychiatry model in devising its data collecting and triage services;

on the other hand, the two systems can come into substantial conflict, since both exercise gate-keeping functions, but for different reasons (Schuster 1995). In many ways, managed care networks are designed to reduce reliance on the PES and even to bypass it in its role of delivering psychiatric emergency care. Networks have emergency phone numbers and 24-hour hotlines for patients to call, and the managed care plan can directly exercise its function of gate-keeping, service authorization, and referral to providers in the plan. These strategies are intended to reduce the need for a participant of the plan to use the PES in an emergency.

It is unclear whether managed care programs lead to an increase or a decrease in the use of PESs. Most managed care is delivered through private insurance providers: health maintenance organizations, preferred provider organizations, and health insurance companies contracting with outside managed care companies. The public entitlement health coverage is also increasingly adopting this model, sometimes contracting with private companies to manage the care or developing their own parallel systems (Stroup and Dorwart 1995). The management of psychiatric care often is "carved out" from general health care (Marshall 1992). In some instances, instituting plans to manage care of the medically ill has resulted in tremendous overuse of PESs. Lazarus (1994) described just such a case, in which there was extensive "dumping" of medically ill patients by redefining them as psychiatric emergencies when the managed care plan was begun. Deficits in managed care systems for the mentally ill can also lead to over-utilization of psychiatric services (Fink and Dubin 1991). One plan had no provision for outpatient psychiatric consultation, hiring only psychologists, social workers, and bachelor's-level therapists to provide outpatient care so as to save money. The affiliated hospital was overwhelmed with admissions because all patients with more difficult cases of mental illness were referred for immediate inpatient care.

Managed care relies on gate-keeping, prior authorization of services, concurrent utilization review, and constraints on choice of providers to attain its goal of cost-effective care. More sophisticated plans provide active case management services. Basic plans restrict admission to contracting hospitals and control utilization by requiring telephone authorization for services. The overall effect has been huge reductions in the use of inpatient psychiatric services and much closer monitoring of the treatment goals and time limits of outpatient treatment. These trends indicate that as managed care expands, the role of the PES should be reduced.

Hillard (1994) examined the balance of these two forces that managed care has exerted on emergency psychiatry and conjectured that in the future the PES will still play a major role in the psychiatric care of managed care patients. Findings from a study of actual managed care patients presenting to a PES (Breslow et al. 1996b) indicated that many of the plan patients visited an emergency service because they had a poor understanding of network procedures or were in too much of a crisis to use them. The majority of managed care patients (65.2%) were not accompanied by family at the time of evaluation, indicating possible deficits in their support system to help them get through the time of crisis. Many (27.5%) were referred to the PES from medical emergency rooms, most probably after overdoses. Some (17.4%) came after coming to the attention of the police, the mobile team, or both. In these cases, the nature of the crisis situation overwhelmed the ability to use network plan procedures. On arrival at the PES, it was not uncommon for these patients (17.4%) to require emergency medication for behavior management. Almost one-half (47.8%) of the plan patients had not utilized their plans to become engaged in outpatient treatment prior to their presentation at the PES. Clearly these are indicators that in the future the role of the PES will continue to be substantial, and further planning of PES services should take into account the need to deal with managed care procedures.

One effect of these procedures is a lengthening of contact time for the managed care patient in the PES (Breslow et al. 1996b). In one study (Breslow et al. 1996b), a greater proportion of managed care patients required extended contact time (26.1%), compared with nonmanaged care patients (17.0%). The contact time for managed care patients may be lengthened by the need to negotiate with the managed care system to obtain approval for hospitalization or outpatient services. Frequently this involves making numerous phone calls. In a typical case, a call may be placed to a reviewer for initial presentation of the patient, and a follow-up call may be needed to obtain the "precertification" for hospitalization. There may then need to be a number of calls placed to find which hospitals in the network have beds and to get the patient approved for admission at one of them. Sometimes additional calls are needed to get approval for ambulance transfer and to alert the receiving service. A major concern is the instance when the two systems come to differing clinical conclusions, in that the emergency service feels that inpatient hospitalization is warranted, but the managed care reviewer denies approval for services. This may make the work of the emergency service especially difficult, because the clinical and legal responsibility for the patient's care remains with the emergency service (Bitterman 1994; Marder 1997). In this case, many more calls may be needed to access higher levels of review within the managed care system.

Sometimes managed care and the PES can work in synergy, with gratifying results and a positive impact on patient care. The origins of managed care plan procedures involve substantial borrowing of the method of approach from the ED triage model. The emphasis is on addressing the immediate problem, assessing risk, and taking action with focused and direct treatment strategies. This is not unlike the way the typical PES staff functions. It is not unusual for staff who were originally trained in the PES or the mobile team to become reviewers for the various managed care plans after leaving the emergency service. This similarity of approach can sometimes help the two systems agree on what is indicated patient care in a given situation. The existence of managed care has been a strong stimulus for the development of extended-evaluation beds and mobile outreach to deal with acute situations while avoiding the use of more expensive systems of care such as inpatient hospitalization. Managed care plans have taken a major role in fostering the development of day hospital programs, which enable the patient to stay in the family but still get the benefits of acute intensive care. This is an important disposition alternative for the PES clinician. The existence of a managed care system can also make the referral work of a PES easier. It helps in obtaining more rapid appointments with private practitioners in the plan.

Many plans utilize a case manager approach. The manager can become a potent ally of the emergency psychiatrist in finding services to maintain the patient in the community. The changing legal situation may promote more partnership and collaboration between the PES and managed care. Court decisions, legislative initiatives, and "patient bill of rights" proposals appear to be extending the legal and clinical responsibility for the patient to the managed care plan, in addition to the already established responsibility of the emergency service.

Teaching

A key advantage of the development of the PES model is the opportunity to have full-time attending psychiatric coverage. This elevates the prestige of the discipline and has changed the whole mind-set with respect to delivering emergency psychiatric care. The organization of a separate service with specialized attending psychiatrists providing the supervision has made it possible to uncover the strengths of the emergency service as a psychiatry teaching setting (Hillard et al. 1993; Thienhaus 1995). The American Association for Emergency Psychiatry (AAEP), consisting of professionals identified primarily with emergency mental health care, serves the "specialty" of emergency psychiatry through its various committees, meetings, and publications. In 1995, the Accreditation Council on Graduate Medical Education required residency programs to provide a supervised experience in a full-time program such as a PES in addition to the service requirements of the "on-call" experience (American Council for Graduate Medical Education 1996). There must be organized instruction and supervised clinical opportunities in emergency psychiatry that lead to the development of knowledge and skills in emergency assessment, crisis management, triage, and evaluation of suicidal patients. The AAEP now offers a model curriculum (Glick et al. 1999).

The PES has many inherent advantages for teaching (Breslow et al. 2000). Services tend to be busy, and the sheer number of patients seen enables the resident to become a "veteran" very quickly. The trainee has a chance to see patients in all stages of psychiatric illness, particularly the acute initial phase, and not just already stabilized patients. The resident or student can gain experience in dealing with first episodes of illness, interpersonal crises, families, and acute substance abuse issues. A tremendous variety of patients present for evaluation. Patients of all ages, socioeconomic groups, and psychiatric diagnoses are seen. There are more opportunities in the emergency service to observe the supervisor conducting interviews and practicing psychiatry than in other settings. The time frame of psychiatric evaluations and the availability of supervising psychiatrists enable a good deal of direct observation of the resident's work as well. The emergency service is an excellent introduction to the mental health system, since it interacts with so many of its elements. The PES must deal with many different referral sources, and this enables trainees to become familiar with the many agencies and systems involved with community care and inpatient services. Many residents have their initial experiences with some current realities of health care financing when they try to get their patient "precertified" for a psychiatric admission. The PES is also frequently at the interface between the medical and psychiatric needs of the patient, enabling the resident to sharpen differential diagnostic skills and medical management.

The primary goal of many services has been the training of psychiatric residents, but the PES can be used to provide an intense and concentrated experience in psychiatry for residents in other specialties such as family practice, internal medicine, and emergency medicine. The flexibility of this setting enables training of many other disciplines as well. At various times, medical students, nursing students, physician's assistants, social work students, and psychology interns have benefitted from exposure to the PES.

Research

The PES plays a major role in psychiatric research that will continue to be important to studies in the future. The most common model for the use of the PES in research is as a source of recruitment and case finding for the research ward or for entry of subjects into outpatient investigations. The development of the PES as a separate service with its own professional staff has led to research directly on the PES itself and on all of its associated services (Breslow 1999). The PES seems, on first view, to be a wonderful resource for psychiatric research, including clinical trials of the effectiveness of treatment alternatives, services research, and outcome studies (Thienhaus 1995). The advantages are the size of the databases, the speed with which data accumulate, and the facility with which collection of data fits in with normal emergency room data gathering.

Alternatively, the nature of the emergency service, with its emphasis on rapid diagnostic assessment, stabilization, and disposition, makes it difficult to control enough variables to carry out detailed studies in this setting. The issues may be formidable in attempting to perform a study of differential treatments and their efficacy in the PES. It is difficult to use rating scales in the PES setting because of high patient acuity, sampling problems, time constraints (i.e., the urgency with which patients must be seen), and resource constraints (e.g., not enough staff to be able to apply the required instruments). Even when experienced staff are available, reliability problems are prevalent in the PES setting. In a study of typical emergency assessment interviews at four different institutions, investigators found poor agreement among experienced psychiatrists concerning key findings such as diagnosis, impulse control, and dangerousness (Way et al. 1998). The issue of patient consent is particularly difficult to resolve because the patient in crisis may, by definition, be unable to give informed consent.

Many research studies regarding the PES and related subjects have appeared in the literature, but it has been difficult to study such services systematically (Breslow et al. 2000). In the past 25 years, there has been an average of between 30 and 40 studies published per year in the field. Services research, descriptive studies, and studies of decision making have been well represented. More work must be done in the study of evaluation, treatments, substance abuse, and special needs populations. It may be that most of the work is done on service aspects and descriptive studies because these are the easiest studies to do and because they can be accomplished in a practical sense. There is a great need for creative approaches to using the strengths of the emergency service as a research setting while compensating for the obvious weaknesses. It is hoped that in the future more resources will become available to use the PES for studying the evaluation process, differential treatments, acute substance abuse, and emergencies in special populations in much greater detail than in the past. This may enable us to move the field forward in finding what does and does not work in emergency psychiatric intervention.

Future Directions

The organization of the PES will continue to develop in the next few decades along the lines that have already been described. There will be an emphasis on separate and more comprehensive services with extended evaluation capacity and the ability to initiate more treatment options. There will be more demand for mobile outreach into the community and crisis residential services as the benefits become more apparent. Efforts to bypass the PES itself and substitute less expensive alternatives may expand as well. Allen (1999) proposed an alternative that maintains the role of the PES but makes it part of a regional system or "consortium model," with a designated center becoming the deliverer of psychiatric emergency care for the whole system. This is similar to the role level 1 trauma centers play in emergency medical care. The advantage is to spread costs over a larger population and allow economies of scale. Whatever happens with these system developments, managed care will continue to have substantial impact on service delivery. The PES will play an ever-growing role as the "filter" for the mental health system with respect to the substance-abusing patient (Breslow et al. 1996a). Underserved populations, such as children, the mentally retarded, and the elderly, will present in increasing numbers.

Technology will continue to transform the emergency service with advances in communication, safety, and computerized records and databases. Cell phones and fax machines have already enabled better communication with the mobile team, increased ability to obtain records, and better coordination of services. Cameras and computerized alarm systems have permitted better safety on the unit. One past effort that has considerable ongoing potential for the future is the development of a computerized telephone logging system for all phone calls that come into the PES. The PES gets many calls concerning emergencies in the community, such as the case of the suicidal patient calling for help. Calls could be coded by the caller, the respondent, the subject of the call, a classification of the emergency level of the call, and the response provided. Such a system has obvious advantages in ensuring good record keeping in a high-risk area, tracking what has happened, aggregating data, and establishing a way to flag problems. This is an area in which many refinements can be applied to the system to ease paperwork burdens, help gain access to information from prior calls, and create a system of "alerts" for staff to know which calls represent true emergencies.

The computerized record can be used in a fashion similar to the phone log to serve as a prompt to the staff of all areas in which information collection is required. PES record keeping can lead to an overflow of old charts that overwhelms the available space, taking room resources that could be better utilized for clinical care. A successful computerized record for the PES could substantially alleviate this problem. The system design would include ease of entry of screening material and ready retrieval of prior entries. Computer "shells" organize the relevant material of the outline for the emergency psychiatric evaluation, including all needed risk assessments. An alerts section that flags areas of special risk with each particular patient should be built in to this outline. This section should be readily available and easily retrieved at the outset of each evaluation. Part of the design could include easy access to all the old records on the patient, but there may be some provision for streamlining the record so the evaluator does not get information overload. A mechanism can be built in to a more sophisticated system to allow "calling up" just the crucial information from the past records relating to past suicide episodes or violence toward others. For example, if suicide evaluation is a particular area of focus, it should be possible to bring up all references to suicide in the prior entries for that patient. Workstations must be readily available to staff so they do not have to wait long to input and retrieve the clinical information that they need.

A vital tool in the future for the PES will be the emergency service database. Many computer software packages are now available that make it a relatively easy task to set up data files and to enter variables into the files. The development of a database of clinical and demographic variables for the patients who visit the PES has been crucial for the organization of the service. It permits tracking of what transpires in the PES to make improvements and facilitates research on important questions about service delivery. Originally, patient contacts were recorded only in a database that the hospital keeps for those admitted to the hospital. However, this left out patients who were not admitted and many variables that were of unique importance to the PES. In developing a database designed for PES use, a key strategy was to select for inclusion only the most relevant, easily scored, and most reliable variables, such as date of visit, patient identification, age, sex, diagnosis, county, and disposition. Otherwise, the whole process would have become too cumbersome and staff would have tended to fall hopelessly behind in data entry. In the database, groups of patients could be aggregated to answer interesting questions about PES functioning. How many patients are being seen in a given period of time? What percentage have bipolar diagnoses? Has the number of children presenting increased? Are patients moving from one county to another? New variables can be added as problems arise. For example, time of arrival, time seen, and time discharged could be added when waiting time for patients becomes a particular area of concern. Addition of new variables, increased staffing to improve data entry, and better staff training to allow routine scoring of rating scales as part of the database could further improve the usefulness of the database to the PES.

An important new trend is the capacity to integrate databases from different areas to improve assessment and treatment. In the future, it may be possible to integrate the PES database with the pharmacy database to help make emergency medication decisions. Other databases could contribute by giving information on substance abuse history, criminal history, and past history of high-risk behavior. As in other areas of American society, this ability to search, and perhaps even combine, databases collected in many diverse areas will undoubtedly raise some complex issues of consent and potential invasion of privacy. The PES psychiatrist will have to be keenly aware of the balance between getting adequate information to manage the risk that the patient may pose to self or others and the need to protect the individual's right to confidentiality and autonomy.

The direction in organization and use of emergency services is toward development of more comprehensive services using the PES model. There are significant advances emerging in communication, safety, computerized records, and databases. This raises the possibility that the emergency psychiatrist of the future will have some wonderful new tools to perform the psychiatric evaluation, initiate treatment, and manage risk for the community.

References

Allen MH: Definitive treatment in the psychiatric emergency service. Psychiatr Q 67:247–262, 1996

Allen MH: Level 1 psychiatric emergency services. Psychiatr Clin North Am 22:713–734, 1999

Allen MH, Currier GW, Hughes DH, et al: The Expert Consensus Guideline Series: treatment of behavioral emergencies. Postgraduate Medicine Special Report. May 2001, pp 1–90

American Council for Graduate Medical Education: Program requirements for residency training in psychiatry, in Graduate Medical Education Directory. 1996–1997. Chicago, IL, American Council for Graduate Medical Education, 1996

Barton GM: A hospital's political environment and its effect on the patient's admission. Hosp Community Psychiatry 25:156–169, 1974

Baxter S, Chodorkoff B, Underhill R: Psychiatric emergencies: dispositional determinants and the validity of the decision to admit. Am J Psychiatry 124:1542–1546, 1968

Bell G, Reinstein DZ, Rajiyah G, et al: Psychiatric screening of admissions to an accident and emergency ward. Br J Psychiatry 158:554–557, 1991

Bengelsdorf H, Alden DC: A mobile crisis unit in the psychiatric emergency room. Hosp Community Psychiatry 38:662–665, 1987

Bitterman RA: Dealing with managed care under COBRA, Parts I and II. Emergency Physician Legal Bulletin 7(4, 5), 1994

Blais A, Georges J: Psychiatric emergencies in a general hospital outpatient department. Can Psychiatr Assoc J 14:123–133, 1969

Breslow RE: A decade of research in a psychiatric emergency service. Emergency Psychiatry 5:32–34, 1999

Breslow RE, Klinger BI, Erickson BJ: Crisis hospitalization on a psychiatric emergency service. Gen Hosp Psychiatry 15:307–315, 1993

Breslow RE, Klinger BI, Erickson BJ: Crisis hospitalization in a psychiatric emergency service. New Dir Ment Health Serv 67:5–12, 1995

Breslow RE, Klinger BI, Erickson BJ: Acute intoxication and substance abuse among patients presenting to a psychiatric emergency service. Gen Hosp Psychiatry 18:183–191, 1996a

Breslow RE, Klinger BI, Erickson BJ: Characteristics of managed care patients in a psychiatric emergency service. Psychiatr Serv 47:1259–1261, 1996b

Breslow RE, Klinger BI, Erickson BJ: Trends in the psychiatric emergency service in the 1990s. Emergency Psychiatry 2:4, 1996c

Breslow RE, Klinger BI, Erickson BJ: Time study of psychiatric emergency service evaluations. Gen Hosp Psychiatry 19:1–4, 1997

Breslow RE, Klinger BI, Erickson BJ: County drift: a type of geographic mobility of chronic psychiatric patients. Gen Hosp Psychiatry 20:44–47, 1998

Breslow RE, Klinger BI, Erickson BJ: The disruptive behavior disorders in the psychiatric emergency service. Gen Hosp Psychiatry 21:214–219, 1999

Breslow RE, Erickson BJ, Cavanaugh KC: The psychiatric emergency service: where we've been and where we're going. Psychiatr Q 71:101–121, 2000

Brodsky L, Pieczynski B: The use of antidepressants in a psychiatric emergency department. J Clin Psychopharmacol 5:35–38, 1985

Buckley RA: Emergency psychiatry: differentiating medical and psychiatric illness. Psychiatric Annals 24:584–591, 1994

Chiu TL, Primeau C: A psychiatric mobile crisis unit in New York City: description and assessment. Int J Soc Psychiatry 37:251–258, 1991

Cohen N, Putnam J, Sullivan A: The mentally ill homeless: isolation and adaptation. Hosp Community Psychiatry 35:922–924, 1984

Commission on Emergency Medical Services: Categorization of hospital emergency capabilities. Chicago, IL, American Medical Association, 1971

Commission on Emergency Medical Services: Provisional guidelines for the optimal categorization of hospital emergency capabilities. Chicago, IL, American Medical Association, 1982

Comstock B: Psychiatric emergency intensive care. Psychiatr Clin North Am 6:305–316, 1983

Currier GW: Atypical antipsychotic medications in the psychiatric emergency service. J Clin Psychiatry 61 (suppl 14):21–26, 2000

Dhossche DM: Suicidal behavior in psychiatric emergency room patients. South Med J 93:310–314, 2000

Elangovan N, Berman S, Meinzer A: Substance abuse among patients presenting at an inner-city psychiatric emergency room. Hosp Community Psychiatry 44:782–784, 1993

Fields S, Weisman GK: Crisis residential treatment: an alternative to hospitalization. New Dir Ment Health Serv 67:23–31, 1995

Fink PH, Dubin WR: No free lunch: limitations on psychiatric care in HMO's. Hosp Community Psychiatry 42:363–365, 1991

Fisher WH, Geller JL, Wirth-Cauchon J: Empirically assessing the impact of mobile crisis capacity on state hospital admissions. Community Ment Health J 26:245–253, 1990

Forster P, King J: Definitive treatment of patients with severe mental disorder in an emergency service, Part I. Hosp Community Psychiatry 45:867–869, 1994a

Forster P, King J: Definitive treatment of patients with severe mental disorder in an emergency service, Part II. Hosp Community Psychiatry 45:1177–1178, 1994b

Freemantle N, House A, Song F, et al: Prescribing selective serotonin reuptake inhibitors as strategy for prevention of suicide. Br Med J 309:249–253, 1994

Geller JL, Fisher WH, McDermeit M: A national survey of mobile crisis services and their evaluation. Psychiatr Serv 46:893–897, 1995

Gerson S, Bassuk E: Psychiatric emergencies: an overview. Am J Psychiatry 137:1–11, 1980

Gillig PM: The spectrum of mobile outreach and its role in the emergency service. New Dir Ment Health Serv 67:13–21, 1995

Gillig PM, Hillard JR, Bell J, et al: The psychiatric emergency service holding area: effect on utilization of inpatient resources. Am J Psychiatry 146:369–372, 1989

Gillig PM, Dumaine M, Hillard JR: Whom do mobile crisis services serve? Hosp Community Psychiatry 41:804–805, 1990

Glick RL: Initiation of antidepressant medications in the emergency setting. Psychiatric Annals 30:251–257, 2000

Glick RL, Allen MH, Brasch J, et al: Guidelines for resident training in emergency psychiatry. Presented at the annual meeting of the American Association of Directors of Psychiatry Residency Training, Los Angeles, CA, 1999

Goodwin R, Lyons JS: An emergency housing program as an alternative to inpatient treatment for persons with severe mental illness. Psychiatr Serv 52:92–95, 2001

Granovetter B: The use of home visits to avoid hospitalization in a psychiatric case. Hosp Community Psychiatry 26:645–646, 1975

Guo S, Biegel DE, Johnsen JA, et al: Assessing the impact of community-based mobile crisis services in preventing hospitalization. Psychiatr Serv 52:223–228, 2001

Hankoff LD, Mischorr MT, Tomlinson KE: A program of crisis intervention in the emergency medical setting. Am J Psychiatry 131:47–50, 1974

Hillard JR: The past and future of psychiatric emergency services in the U.S. Hosp Community Psychiatry 45:541–543, 1994

Hillard JR, Zitek B, Thienhaus OJ: Residency training in emergency psychiatry. Acad Psychiatry 17:125–129, 1993

Hirschfeld RMA, Allen MH, McEvoy J, et al: Safety and tolerability of oral loading divalproex sodium in acutely manic bipolar patients. J Clin Psychiatry 60:815–818, 1999

Hockberger RS, Binder LS, Graber MA, et al: The model of the clinical practice of emergency medicine. Ann Emerg Med 37:745–770, 2001

Hu SC: Computerized monitoring of emergency department patient flow. Am J Emerg Med 11:8–11, 1993

Hughes DH: Trends and treatment models in emergency psychiatry. Hosp Community Psychiatry 44:927–928, 1993

Ianzito BM, Fine J, Sprague B, et al: Overnight admission for psychiatric emergencies. Hosp Community Psychiatry 29:728–730, 1978

Jarvis E: On the supposed increase of insanity. American Journal of Insanity 8:334–364, 1851

Johnson S, Thornicroft G: Emergency psychiatric services in England and Wales. Br Med J 311:287–288, 1995

Kane BL, Kelly K, Petro J: Implementing an extended crisis evaluation unit in the emergency department in response to New Jersey screening law. J Emerg Nurs 19:426–430, 1993

Kapur S, Mieczkowski T, Mann JJ: Antidepressant medications and the relative risk of suicide attempt and suicide. JAMA 268:3441–3445, 1992

Kates N, Eaman S, Santone J, et al: An integrated regional emergency psychiatry service. Gen Hosp Psychiatry 18:251–256, 1996

Lamb HR, Lamb DM: A nonhospital alternative to acute hospitalization. Hosp Community Psychiatry 35:728–730, 1984

Lazarus A: Dumping psychiatric patients in the managed care sector. Hosp Community Psychiatry 45:529–530, 1994

Marder D: Hospital policy: responding to COBRA. Emergency Psychiatry 3:31–33, 1997

Marshall PE: The mental health HMO: capitation funding for the chronically mentally ill. Community Ment Health J 28:111–120, 1992

McClelland PA: The emergency psychiatric system. Psychiatr Clin North Am 6:225–232, 1983

Merson S, Tyrer P, Onyett S, et al: Early intervention in psychiatric emergencies: a controlled clinical trial. Lancet 339:1311–1324, 1992

Mosher L, Menn A: Soteria: an alternative to hospitalization for schizophrenics. Current Psychiatric Therapy 21:189–203, 1982

Munizza C, Furlan P, d'Elia A, et al: Emergency psychiatry: a review of the literature. Acta Psychiatr Scand 374:1–51, 1993

Oldham JM, DeMasi ME: An integrated approach to emergency psychiatric care. New Dir Ment Health Serv 67:33–42, 1995

Oldham JM, Lin A, Breslin L: Comprehensive psychiatric emergency services. Psychiatr Q 61:57–66, 1990

Rae RP: Level system for psychiatric emergency care. Emergency Psychiatry 3:52–53, 1997

Rhine MW, Mayerson P: Crisis hospitalization within a psychiatric emergency service. Am J Psychiatry 127:1386–1391, 1971

Rubinstein D: Re-hospitalization versus family crisis intervention. Am J Psychiatry 129:715–720, 1972

Ruiz P, Vazquez W, Vazquez K: The mobile unit: a new approach in mental health. Community Ment Health J 9:18–24, 1973

Saunders CE: Time study of patient movement through the emergency department: sources of delay in relation to patient acuity. Ann Emerg Med 16:1244–1248, 1987

Schneider SM, Hamilton GC, Moyer P, et al: Definition of emergency medicine. Acad Emerg Med 5:348–351, 1998

Schuster JM: Frustration or opportunity? The impact of managed care on emergency psychiatry. New Dir Ment Health Serv 67:101–108, 1995

Soreff S: New directions and added dimensions in home psychiatric treatment. Am J Psychiatry 140:1213–1216, 1983

Stebbins LA, Hardman GL: A survey of psychiatric consultants at a suburban emergency room. Gen Hosp Psychiatry 15:234–242, 1993

Stroul BA: Residential crisis services: a review. Hosp Community Psychiatry 39:1095–1099, 1988

Stroup RS, Dorwart RA: The impact of a managed mental health program on Medicaid recipients with severe mental illness. Psychiatr Serv 46:885–889, 1995

Szuster RR, Schanbacher BL, McCann SC: Underdiagnosis of psychoactive substance induced organic mental disorders in emergency psychiatry. Am J Drug Alcohol Abuse 16:319–327, 1990

Thienhaus OJ: Academic issues in emergency psychiatry. New Dir Ment Health Serv 67:109–114, 1995

Tufnell G, Bouras N, Watson J, et al: Home assessment and treatment in a community psychiatric service. Acta Psychiatr Scand 72:20–28, 1985

Way BB, Allen MH, Mumpower JL, et al: Interrater agreement among psychiatrists in psychiatric emergency assessments. Am J Psychiatry 155:1423–1428, 1998

Weisman G, Feirstein A, Thomas C: Three-day hospitalization: a model for intervention. Arch Gen Psychiatry 21:620–629, 1969

West DA, Litwok E, Oberlander K: Emergency psychiatric home visiting: report of four years' experience. J Clin Psychiatry 41:113–118, 1980

Wingerson D, Russo J, Ries R, et al: Use of psychiatric emergency services and enrollment status in a public managed mental health care plan. Psychiatr Serv 52:1494–1501, 2001

Zealberg JJ, Christie SD, Puckett JA, et al: A mobile crisis program: collaboration between emergency psychiatric services and police. Hosp Community Psychiatry 43:612–615, 1992

Chapter 2

Medical, Psychiatric, and Cognitive Assessment in the Psychiatric Emergency Service

Glenn W. Currier, M.D., M.P.H.
Michael H. Allen, M.D.
Mark R. Serper, Ph.D.
Adam J. Trenton, B.A.
Marc L. Copersino, Ph.D.

The proper assessment of patients presenting to psychiatric emergency services (PESs) is a complex and hotly debated issue. Clinicians working in this arena are expected to recognize and appropriately deal with the gamut of medical, psychiatric, and social reasons for which patients present. These efforts are hampered by a lack of agreed-on screening tools, procedures, protocols, or even expected outcomes. The training and experience of PES personnel differ from setting to setting, and the resources available to staff within each PES also vary widely. Reliance on the medical emergency department (ED) to "own" the medical needs of psychiatric patients has been the norm. However, psychiatric physicians working in a variety of settings have begun to realize the crucial role they play in recognizing and treating physical illness in mentally ill patients. While some PES physicians have been proactive in assuming that role, others have not. As a result, practices vary widely from site to site and from practitioner to practitioner.

In this chapter, we focus on the sparse literature that exists to guide medical, psychiatric, and particularly cognitive assessment in the PES environment. Barriers to consistent practice are identified, and suggested approaches are outlined.

Medical Assessment in the Psychiatric Emergency Service

The evolution of emergency medicine from general medicine is relatively recent. As is the current case in the PES, until the past few decades practitioners in emergency "rooms" often were moonlighters whose main professional duties were elsewhere. As the field of emergency medicine evolved into a distinct medical specialty, striking changes occurred in the philosophy of practice. Emergency medicine physicians began to see their task as isolation and treatment of the presenting condition. Patients who present with a broken bone may get a focused assessment appropriate to that body part, but a more extensive physical examination and medical history may be deferred to the primary care office, assuming there is one.

As of this writing, the ACGME requires that most psychiatry residency programs offer a scant 4 months of general medicine and 2 months of neurology in the internship year. As a result, many psychiatrists are poorly equipped to handle even routine medical problems.

Psychiatrists in emergency settings are thus faced with a dilemma. As emergency medicine has evolved, the tradition of relying on colleagues in the medical ED for "medical clearance" of psychiatric patients is inconsistent with their practice philosophy. Emergency physicians do not conceptualize their role as something as diffuse as "clearance," with no index symptoms to explore. As will be discussed in more detail elsewhere in this chapter, patients receiving care in the PES are increasingly being found to be medically ill, and many of the serious medical comorbidities encountered in people with psychiatric illness may actually be caused by psychiatric treatment (e.g., dystonia). Psychiatrists often are in a better position to recognize and treat these problems.

The PES demands medically competent psychiatrists. To that end, the American Association for Emergency Psychiatry (AAEP) and others have begun to devise structured residency and fellowship curricula to fill the gaps common in general psychiatry residency programs. Grounded in the biopsychosocial model, these curricula stress an integrated approach to mind-body health.

Frequency of Medical Morbidity

Determining exact rates of medical comorbidity in psychiatric patients has been problematic, because several studies did not include control groups, and because the patient cohorts studied varied by age, location, and year of study. However, evidence does suggest that patients with psychiatric disorders commonly present with comorbid medical problems (Table 2–1). Koranyi (1980) reviewed studies conducted over the course of 40 years and determined that of the approximately 4,000 cases reviewed, more than 50% of the patients had major medical illnesses; in approximately 20% of all studies reviewed, the somatic conditions were directly related to psychiatric symptoms. Karasu et al. (1980) examined the prevalence of physical illness among various psychiatric populations and found that 15% of inpatients and 52% of outpatients had medical problems, over half of which were "potentially serious."

Carlson et al. (1981) reported that 140 of 2,000 patients consecutively seen in the PES at Royal Ottawa Hospital presented with physical illness as their only or primary diagnosis. Among 75% of these patients, psychiatric symptoms could be attributed in some way to somatic dysfunction. Collectively, patients with physical complaints were more likely to be over 60 years of age (16%) and to present with alcoholism (24%) or organic brain syndrome (13%) than those without physical problems. The most common physical diagnoses among these patients were extrapyramidal symptoms (19%), overdose (16%), delirium tremens (11%), seizures (5%), and gastrointestinal bleeding (5%). Human immunodeficiency virus (HIV) is also highly prevalent in some mentally ill populations, with rates of 4%–23% reported (Brown and Jemmott 2000).

Table 2–1. Prevalence of medical problems in psychiatric patients

Authors	Type of setting	Number of patients included	Rate of physical illness (%)
Karasu et al. (1980)	Inpatient	612	15
	Outpatient	200	52
Carlson et al. (1981)	PES	200	7
Hall et al. (1981)	Inpatient	100	80
Lima and Pai (1987)	CMHC	427	41
Koran et al. (1989)	Public mental health system	529	38
Olshaker et al. (1997)	ED	345	19

Note. CMHC = community mental health center; ED = emergency department; PES = psychiatric emergency service.

Classification of Physical Diseases as Causative, Exacerbating, or Incidental

In some cases, medical illness directly causes or exacerbates psychiatric symptoms (Table 2–2). The high prevalence of unrecognized physical illness causative of psychiatric symptoms among psychiatric inpatients was documented in several older studies. Knutsen and DuRand (1991) performed extensive medical evaluations of 78 psychiatric inpatients 1–2 weeks after their admission evaluation and found previously unrecognized physical illness in 68 (87%) of the patients. In 3 patients, physical illnesses, including two cases of cerebral atrophy and one instance of adverse effects of medication, were judged to be causative of psychiatric symptoms. Hall et al. (1981) determined that among 100 patients consecutively admitted to a research ward, 46% had an unrecognized medical illness that caused or exacerbated psychiatric symptoms. Of these 46 patients, 28 displayed rapid and significant improvement of psychiatric symptoms after the underlying physical disorders were treated. The types of diseases most frequently judged to be causative of psychiatric symptoms included endocrine disorders (36%), polysystem diseases (18%), hematological disorders (15%), and cardiovascular disorders (8%).

Table 2–2. Medical disorders that commonly cause or exacerbate psychiatric symptoms

Medical/toxic	CNS	Infections	Metabolic/ endocrine	Cardiopulmonary	Miscellaneous
Alcohol and drug abuse	CNS infection	Acute rheumatic fever	Adrenal disease	Arrhythmias	Anemia
Amphetamines	Hypertensive encephalopathy	Hepatitis	Electrolyte imbalances	Asthma	Lupus
Anabolic steroids	Intracranial aneurysm	Pneumonia	Hepatic encephalopathy	Congestive heart failure	NMS
Benzodiazepines	Migraine headache	Sepsis	Renal disease	COPD	Serotonin syndrome
Cocaine	Normal-pressure hydrocephalus	Syphilis	Thyroid disease	Myocardial infarction	Temporal arteritis
Ecstacy	Seizures	Urinary tract infection	Vitamin deficiencies	Pulmonary embolism	Vasculitis
Heroin	Subdural hematoma				
LSD	Tumor				
PCP					
THC					
Prescription drugs (examples)					
Digitalis					
Propranolol					
Seizure drugs					
Steroids					

Note. CNS = central nervous system; COPD = chronic obstructive pulmonary disease; LSD = lysergic acid diethylamide; NMS = neuroleptic malignant syndrome; PCP = phencyclidine; THC = Δ-tetrahydrocannabinol.
Source. Data from Williams and Shepherd 2000.

The presence of medical disorders causative of psychiatric symptoms has also been reported among psychiatric outpatients. Hall et al. (1978) reported on 658 consecutive psychiatric outpatients who received comprehensive medical and laboratory evaluation aided by a symptoms checklist. Medical disorders causative of psychiatric symptoms were discovered in 9.1% of cases. The most common diagnoses among these patients were cardiovascular and endocrine disorders.

In addition to physical illnesses that directly produce psychiatric symptoms, there are many that exacerbate existing mental disorders. It is estimated that somatic conditions are directly related to psychiatric symptoms in 9%–42% of patients presenting for psychiatric services (Koranyi 1980). Neurological dysfunction and nutritional deficiencies may accentuate psychiatric dysfunction. Patients with neurological conditions frequently present with chronic psychiatric syndromes that respond poorly to treatment. Koran et al. (1989) discovered a high prevalence of medical problems among patients seen in a public mental health system. Of the 529 patients who were medically evaluated, 51 presented with diseases that are likely to exacerbate mental illness. The most common problems were organic brain disease (23%), diabetes (20%), and seizures or epilepsy (6%).

In other instances, the presence of somatic disease in an individual with mental illness is largely incidental. A high frequency of incidental medical illness occurs in mentally ill patients because of personal and systematic barriers to adequate health care. A large proportion of patients with mental illnesses do not view their physical health as a priority, may be noncompliant with recommended care, and may have a negative self-image, which may lead them to accept inadequate health care coverage (Lieberman and Coburn 1986).

Further obstacles occur as mentally ill patients attempt to interact with the health care system. The physical and mental health care received by these patients is often fragmentary in nature, and thus comorbid diagnoses may be overlooked. Medical providers may be reluctant to treat chronically mentally ill patients, who may be Medicaid recipients, inarticulate, substance abusing, and poorly kempt (Lieberman and Coburn 1986).

Patients with schizophrenia may be at particular risk. Lima and Pai (1987) reported on 358 cases of active schizophrenia among patients in a poor, inner-city population; 38% of these patients were diagnosed with one or more physical problems. The most common diagnoses among these patients were hypertension (35%), diabetes (19%), obesity (13%), asthma or bronchitis (13%), seizures (8%), and orthopedic injury (7%).

Sensitivity and Efficiency of Diagnostic Procedures

To date, a consistent protocol for medical evaluation in the PES has not been established, though several methods of evaluation have been used, with varying results. In many cases, the only method of screening for physical illness is a cursory medical history. Henneman et al. (1994) evaluated 100 consecutive patients seen in an urban PES, 63 of whom were determined to have an organic basis to their illness. However, only 27% of patients related a medical history indicative of significant physical illness. Olshaker et al. (1997) evaluated 345 patients seen in the ED of an urban teaching hospital, noting medical problems in 65 patients (19%). In this retrospective study, the medical history alone identified all relevant physical illnesses in 94% of cases. The authors concluded that vital signs and a basic history and physical were adequate and that universal laboratory and toxicology screening was of low yield. In some cases, cognitive limitations of patients or poor cooperation may compromise the reliability of medical histories. Still, this process is a critical initial step in the process of medical screening.

Vital signs should be obtained when a patient presents to a medical or psychiatric ED. Olshaker et al. (1997) indicated that taking vital signs had a sensitivity of 17% for detecting medical illnesses among patients receiving psychiatric services.

Physical examinations are sometimes performed with patients in the PES; in one study (Olshaker et al. 1997), physical exams were reported to have a sensitivity of 51% for detecting current medical problems. However, Henneman et al. (1994) reported significant findings on the basis of a physical exam in 6 of

100 patients that would not have been detected by history alone, though 63 of these patients had diseases of organic etiology. Other authors highlight the usefulness of physical examinations in psychiatric patients with obvious or known medical comorbidity (Viner et al. 1996).

Obtaining "labs" poses a financial and time burden for both patients and the system as a whole. Some services rely on a standard battery of laboratory tests, applied rote to each patient regardless of presenting complaint. This approach is problematic for several reasons. In the absence of a clinical indication, laboratory tests may result in significant "false positive" results, subjecting the patient to needless follow-up examinations. Olshaker et al. (1997) reported that laboratory tests detected significant medical issues in approximately 20% of patients, but only a small minority of these would not have been detected in the history and physical.

Other authors advocate more extensive and invasive evaluation for alert patients presenting with new-onset psychiatric complaints. Henneman et al. (1994) noted that two-thirds of 100 such patients had an organic etiology. These authors recommended the following: history and physical examination; alcohol and drug screens; electrolytes; BUN (blood urea nitrogen); creatinine; glucose; calcium; CPK (creatine phosphokinase), if urine dipstick is positive for blood without red blood cells (RBCs) on microscopic examination; cranial computed tomography (CT); and lumbar puncture if other tests were not conclusive. The findings of this small study may relate to the unique population served at that setting: most PESs find this elaborate protocol impractical and unnecessary.

Urine or serum toxicology is a potentially useful tool in the PES because many individuals with mental illness have comorbid substance abuse problems. There are three situations in which toxicology screens are suggested: 1) if a patient has recently been exposed to poisonous substances, 2) if clinical data suggest recent drug or alcohol use, or 3) if there is suspicion of circulating drug levels outside of the therapeutic range (Thienhaus 1992). In one study, 29% of patients showed definitive positive test results on alcohol and drug screening (Henneman et al.

1994). Olshaker et al. (1997) noted that of 345 patients, 90 and 214 tested positive for alcohol and illicit drugs, respectively. However, many of these patients readily admitted to substance abuse. In all, self-reporting indicated an 88% positive predictive value for drug use and a 73% positive predictive value for ethanol use (Olshaker et al. 1997). In the ED environment, it may be practical to use qualitative tests to determine the presence or absence of alcohol or illicit drugs in the blood or urine. Qualitative tests are less expensive and more expedient than standard quantitative screening methods (Thienhaus 1992).

Other diagnostic procedures are less frequently warranted for PES patients. Henneman et al. (1994) performed a CT scan in 82 patients and found significant abnormalities in 8. The lumbar puncture was suggested by these authors for patients presenting with new and rapidly worsening mental status changes, though the results are rarely positive. Tests of liver may be helpful in cases of delirium, alcohol abuse, or suspected hepatic impairment, especially if these tests are done prior to starting hepatically metabolized medications. Thyroid function tests may be helpful, particularly in the context of mood disorders (Thienhaus 1992).

Routine electrocardiographic screening has not been the norm in most settings. Hollister (1995) reported that blanket screening is not indicated unless the patients are over 50 years of age, have a known cardiac condition, or are treated with a drug known to increase cardiac conduction times. The introduction of newer atypical antipsychotics known to prolong QT_C intervals may increase the need for routine electrocardiographic testing.

The American College of Emergency Physicians (1999) has recently published a clinical policy on the initial approach to patients with altered mental status that provides excellent guidance on the appropriateness of various diagnostic studies.

Triage

Patients with urgent psychiatric complaints generally present to the PES via a medical emergency department. Prior to referral to PES, patients undergo varying degrees of medical evaluation. The first contact a psychiatric patient generally has with medical staff occurs at triage. At this point the process of determining whether psychiatric complaints are "functional" or organic in nature is initiated. Making this distinction is a daunting task; for example, many neurological dysfunctions (e.g., subcortical dysrhythmias and elliptogenic discharge) can present as psychiatric symptoms.

To begin ruling out various etiologies, triage personnel can obtain primary screening data. A basic medical history can be obtained to determine if the patient is aware of any physical problems. In attaining a medical history, the triage staff should inquire about the presence of cardiovascular, pulmonary, rheumatological, metabolic/endocrine, neurological, and oncological problems. The triage nurse (or clinician if not a nurse) or other staff should also inquire about recent illness, current medications, infection, trauma, or surgery. Vital signs, including pulse, respiratory rate, temperature, and blood pressure, should be taken initially. If one of the vital signs is outside of the normal range, an organic etiology should at least be suspected (Thienhaus 1992; Williams and Shepherd 2000). Orthostatic changes can be a side effect of anticholinergic medications, an indication of diabetes, or a symptom of alcohol withdrawal or other causes of volume depletion (Hatta et al. 1998). A brief mental status examination is useful, with particular attention paid to findings suggestive of delirium (Kaufman and Zun 1995). Additionally, a report of the patient's appearance with regard to attention, affect, dress, grooming, and hygiene may be helpful (Williams and Shepherd 2000).

If, at this point, the primary etiology is considered to be a functional psychiatric disorder, the patient would likely be referred to a mental health practitioner. If the primary etiology is judged to be organic, a more comprehensive physical examination should be performed. This is particularly true if mental status symptoms suggest delirium in the differential diagnosis. Elderly patients with acute changes in mental status should also be given a physical examination and urinalysis to screen for acute infection (Thienhaus 1992).

Although there are situations in which a physical examination is clearly indicated, the proper location for such an examination has been debated. One perspective is that a physical should be performed in the PES by a psychiatrist, since he or she has been trained to distinguish organic causes of psychiatric symptoms from functional psychiatric disorders. More commonly, continued physical evaluation is performed in the medical ED, and transfer to the PES occurs after medical clearance.

Medical Clearance

Medical clearance is a loosely defined term that is commonly used to indicate that a patient is physically stable and can be transferred to psychiatry without immediate deterioration. This term is commonly used in three related scenarios. Medical clearance may be given if no physical illness is thought to be present in a patient with psychiatric complaints. It may also be applied to a patient who has a known comorbid illness that is not thought to be the primary cause of the presenting psychiatric symptoms. Finally, medical clearance may indicate that a patient's medical condition no longer requires medical treatment and that he or she is stable for transfer to psychiatric services (Williams and Shepherd 2000).

Comprehensive medical clearance may include medical history, a physical examination, vital signs, laboratory tests, and radiography (Korn et al. 2000). Depending on the patient's condition, a focused physical examination may be performed.

Assessments of attention and cognition can be useful in determining whether or not a psychiatric disorder is responsible for the presenting problem. The head may be examined for trauma or evidence of prior surgery. An ocular examination can be indicated if illicit drug use is suspected. Pinpoint pupils are a classic sign of narcotic use, though poisonings, overdoses, or metabolic abnormalities may also explain them. Dilated pupils can indicate intoxication with lysergic acid diethylamide (LSD), sympathomimetic drugs, or anticholinergic drugs; withdrawal from sedative-hypnotic agents; or postaxonic injury (Williams and Shepherd 2000). Examination of the neck usually involves observation of range of motion and palpation of the thyroid gland (Thienhaus 1992). Abnormalities include meningeal signs, thyroid enlargement, and nodules, among other features (Williams and Shepherd 2000). Inspection and auscultation of the chest are also important, because many cardiovascular and pulmonary deficits can present with psychiatric symptoms (Thienhaus 1992; Williams and Shepherd 2000). Abdominal cavity problems such as obstruction, perforation, hemorrhage, and infection may also alter mental status (Williams and Shepherd 2000). Both a brief neurological examination, documenting cranial nerve functioning, deep tendon reflexes, motor status, cerebellar function (including tremor), and balance, and an inspection of eyes are essential (Thienhaus 1992).

Laboratory tests should be ordered on the basis of findings obtained in the physical evaluation, medical history, or review of systems. Some laboratory tests performed in the PES for specific indications include electrolytes, pulse oximetry, electrocardiography thyroid function tests, B_{12}/folate levels, lead level, syphilis serology, carboxyhemoglobin level, antinuclear antibody, liver panel, renal panel, complete blood count (CBC), blood sugar, urinalysis, chest X ray, serum osmolarity, and ammonia level (Thienhaus 1992; Williams and Shepherd 2000). The threshold for laboratory tests should be reduced for patients with new-onset psychiatric symptoms and for those in the youngest and oldest age brackets (Williams and Shepherd 2000).

Physicians in emergency medicine and psychiatry must gauge the utility of procedures against the associated costs. Riba and Hale (1990) reviewed 5,005 patients seen in an emergency room; 123 of the patients complained chiefly of psychiatric symptoms. There was significant variation in the thoroughness of the medical evaluation that these patients received. The following assessments were relatively regularly performed: checking vital signs (68%), noting general appearance (36%), and recording the history of presenting illness (33%). The tendency to assess specific organ systems varied, with heart (64%), HEENT (head, ears, eyes, nose, throat) (63%), and lung (60%) examinations being the most common. Significant medical findings were discovered in 16 patients (12%), with the most common being hypertension (9 patients), tachycardia (4), and diabetes mellitus (3).

Korn et al. (2000) examined the utility of comprehensive medical clearance in the ED. A total of 212 patients who presented with a psychiatric complaint and required a psychiatric evaluation before discharge were included in the study. Eighty patients presented with isolated psychiatric complaints associated with past psychiatric history. None of these patients showed abnormalities on laboratory or radiographic assessment. The remaining 132 patients presented with medically based chief complaints or past medical history requiring further evaluation. These complaints correlated with the need for laboratory and radiographic evaluation. Korn et al. concluded that patients with a past psychiatric history, negative physical findings, and stable vital signs who deny current medical problems may be referred to psychiatric services without additional testing in the ED.

Various attempts have been made to create a standard physical examination for patients with psychiatric complaints (Riba and Hale 1990). Summers et al. (1981a, 1981b) devised an abbreviated physical examination designed specifically for psychiatric patients. This protocol detected a high number of unsuspected physical abnormalities—an average of 5.3 new findings per patient. Sox et al. (1989) developed a medical algorithm for assessing physical disease in psychiatric patients. This method, which employs a six-node assessment tool that incorporates aspects of medical history, laboratory tests, vital signs, and other factors, was determined to successfully detect medical problems in 90% of physically ill patients.

Focused Assessment

Although it is important to use discretion in performing clinical evaluations and diagnostic procedures, it is also critical to avoid overlooking important physical diagnoses. Because EDs are generally busy, there is commonly a tendency to focus only on the presenting complaint, despite the existence of other potentially exacerbating physical problems. As a result, patients with psychiatric complaints may be referred to the PES without receiving sufficient physical assessment.

Tintinalli et al. (1994) examined the prevalence of missed physical diagnoses among 298 patients presenting to an ED with psychiatric complaints. Among the patients in whom medical disease should have been identified, 80% were designated as medically clear. Though mental status is considered to be an important indication of the nature of psychiatric complaints, a mental status examination was not performed at triage with 56% of these patients. Significant process deficiencies were commonly found in neurological examinations. Consequently, many patients were admitted to inpatient psychiatric units with undiagnosed medical illnesses.

Comorbid medical illness escaping diagnosis in the ED is particularly problematic in special populations, including the geriatric population and among patients with organic brain syndromes. Many of these patients are referred to the PES without a physical examination, despite the fact that both groups are at an increased risk for having a medical illness. Waxman et al. (1984) examined the care received in emergency services by middle-aged and elderly patients presenting with organic brain syndromes or psychiatric dysfunction. Among patients with organic brain syndromes in both age groups, significant assessment deficiencies were noted; for example, 27 of 58 patients received no pulmonary examination, 33 of 58 patients did not receive a chest radiograph, and 40 of 58 patients did not have an electrocardiogram (ECG). In 23 of 58 patients, there was a lack of clinical chemistry. Among patients who did receive these tests, a high incidence of positive results—for example, 7 of 13 patients who received chest radiographs and 7 of 19 who received a CBC—was discovered.

Protocols for providing physical examinations in the PES vary among programs, with some including a medical evaluation as part of standard overall assessment and others providing evaluation only when patients are admitted to the hospital or when the PES sees a specific indication. Schuster et al. (1996) compared two emergency psychiatric programs with different approaches to medical assessment. At Allegheny General Hospital, patients presenting to the PES received a physical examination as a matter of standard procedure, whereas at the University of Cincinnati Hospital, patients received physical examination only after admission to a psychiatric unit or if the psychiatrist in the emergency room specifically requested it. Only 5 of 360 patients in either setting were transferred to a medical service after admission to a psychiatric unit.

Personnel Qualifications

PES psychiatrists must be competent to screen for serious causal or contributory illness. Ideally, they should be capable of caring for incidental medical problems as well. As the health care system has changed, psychiatrists have been given additional responsibilities in terms of delivering primary care services. However, it is unclear whether psychiatrists receive sufficient primary care training. On graduating from medical school, some psychiatrists may complete an internship similar to their colleagues in medicine. However, beyond this point, primary care training tends to be limited, unless fellowship training is pursued. Psychiatric residencies are only required to incorporate 4 months of primary care experience and 2 months of neurology. Kick et al. (1997) recommended that a wider range of medical experiences—including supervision from a psychiatrist with expertise in medical contributions to psychiatric presentations and treatment—be incorporated into residency programs.

Although psychiatrists may not receive comprehensive training in all facets of general medicine, they are generally qualified to address pathologies with which patients commonly present in the PES. In some cases, however, social workers serve as the primary psychiatric consultants to emergency services (Wallace et al. 1985). In general, these social workers are given some background on biomedical issues pertinent to psychiatric treatment, but organic causes of psychiatric disorders may go unnoticed, with catastrophic consequences.

Some question whether psychiatrists are the appropriate providers to treat primary medical disorders. Golomb et al. (2000) assembled a panel of psychiatrists, internists, and other medical specialists to address this issue. In most cases, the panel regarded a psychiatrist, with support available from an internist, as an appropriate treatment provider. The entire panel agreed that a psychiatrist would be an appropriate treatment provider for 45% of screening and preventive counseling indications. Moreover, a simple consensus indicated that a psychiatrist would be an appropriate treatment provider for 11 of the 13 most common reasons for ambulatory care, including hypertension and stomach pain (Golomb et al. 2000).

Carney et al. (1998) examined the level of knowledge and attitudes of psychiatrists toward delivering preventive medical care. Residents and faculty in psychiatry and general internal medicine were asked to complete a questionnaire, which included 20 case scenarios that assessed baseline knowledge of clinical and preventive services. Despite their lack of specific training in these matters, psychiatrists exhibited a relatively strong knowledge of preventive medical services. Moreover, they acknowledged the importance of these services and expressed interest in their delivery.

Psychiatric Assessment in the Psychiatric Emergency Service

Types of Assessment

The scope of assessment performed in PESs may vary greatly, depending on the nature of the institution. Generally, psychiatric assessment in the PES serves three primary functions. A disposition must be determined rapidly, since a patient most often may be detained in an ED only for up to 24 hours. Disposition typically involves referring a patient to low-intensity outpatient care or admitting the patient to an inpatient unit. A second function of the PES is to determine whether patients require involuntary civil commitment, a complex decision based on clinical as well as legal factors. A third function of assessment in the PES, applicable in some situations, is to reach a definitive diagnosis so that proper treatment can be initiated.

Determining an appropriate disposition is a central role of the PES. Some literature suggests that a systematic approach should be applied to the formation of a disposition on the basis of specific diagnostic and patient variables. In a retrospective analysis of patients who presented to an acute care psychiatric hospital,

Rabinowitz et al. (1995) noted that certain case features were predictive of specific dispositions. Factors predictive of hospitalization included three or more prior hospitalizations, psychosis, suicidal behavior as the presenting complaint, involuntarily presentation, and low Global Assessment of Functioning (GAF) scores. An increased likelihood of being placed on a locked unit was associated with age being between 20 and 30, being a danger to self or others, being male, having a low GAF score, and having a diagnosis of nonorganic psychosis. Patients who were discharged after a brief stay in the emergency service were likely to display suicidal ideation as a presenting problem, have a GAF ranging from 31 to 50, and carry a diagnosis of a personality disorder. In this sample, levels of psychopathology and dangerousness to self or others were primary predictors of disposition.

Way and Banks (2001) examined factors predictive of admission and release decisions in four urban PES programs. A total of 465 patients were assessed on 10 clinical dimensions, including depression and psychosis, as well as five additional variables (i.e., age, sex, ethnicity, diagnosis, and previous inpatient admission). Among the variables assessed, five (level of danger to self, severity of psychosis, ability to care for self, impulse control, and severity of depression) were judged to be significantly indicative of admission or release. This five-factor model was able to account for 51.2% of the variance in case disposition and correctly classify 84.4% of cases.

While a number of clinical considerations are involved in determining a patient's disposition, the decision to detain involuntarily a patient incorporates additional complexities, including local legislation. Segal et al. (2001) noted that 109 of 583 patients (18.7%) seen in the PES of a California general hospital were retained against their wishes. Involuntary admission is contingent on a patient's presenting with acute dangerousness to self or others, both of which may be difficult to assess in a relatively brief period. Segal et al. (1988a) formulated a systematic measure of dangerousness, called Three Ratings of Involuntary Admissibility (TRIAD), to aid in the interpretation of civil commitment standards. TRIAD consists of three checklists, comprising a total of 88 questions. It was designed to simulate clinical judgment by scoring patterns of behavior and circumstance as more or less dangerous. Among the 251 patients evaluated by Segal et al. (1988a), TRIAD correctly predicted disposition in 76% of cases.

In the current legal environment, dangerousness may have a greater influence on civil commitment than does need for treatment. As a result, more severely mentally ill patients may be neglected in favor of those who present with a propensity for dangerous behavior. However, Segal et al. (1988b) noted that among 198 patients seen in five different psychiatric emergency departments, those rated as most dangerous on TRIAD were also the most severely mentally ill. In addition to the positive significant correlation found between dangerousness and major mental disorders, dangerousness was also significantly related to the severity of certain symptoms, such as impulsivity. Consequently, patients who were retained were more likely to show impulsivity (92%) than patients who were released (38%). However, there was no apparent relationship between dangerousness and Axis II personality disorders. In a follow-up report, Segal et al. (1988c) noted that a combination of dangerousness and the presence of a mental disorder predicted disposition for 93% of new patients and 88% of recurrent patients.

There has been some speculation in the field that factors apart from diagnostic considerations may influence a clinician's decision to hospitalize a patient. To address this issue, Segal et al. (2001) examined various aspects of procedural justice related to the involuntary retention of patients seen in the psychiatric EDs of California general hospitals. The purpose of this analysis was to determine whether evaluation was carried out in a manner that would lead an impartial observer to believe that admissions decisions were based solely on legal criteria. Four clinical admissions criteria were analyzed: the assignment of a DSM-III diagnosis of a psychotic disorder, the patient's performance on the TRIAD scale, the likelihood that the patient could be successfully treated, and the capacity of the patient to benefit from hospitalization. Segal et al. also examined institutional constraints and social bias indicators that might have contributed to a clinician's selection of a coercive disposition. It was concluded that most clinicians relied primarily on appropriate admission criteria in making decisions to retain patients, thus promoting procedural justice in civil commitment.

However, Engleman et al. (1998) found that clinical as well as system variables were relevant. In their study, a risk assessment questionnaire was completed for 169 patients who presented to a community mental health center with some perceived degree of risk. Danger to self and substantial inability to perform self-care were both strong predictors of the overall risk rating, which was in turn significantly associated with the decision to detain patients. Three underlying constructs, not directly related to clinical factors, were also associated with the decision to detain patients: the clinician's detention ratio (i.e., the proportion of patients detained by the clinician in the past 3 months), the availability of detention beds in the community, and the setting in which the evaluation occurred (i.e., emergency service or mobile crisis). Predictably, clinicians with generally greater inclination to admit patients continued this trend during the study period. Clinicians were collectively more likely to admit patients when beds in the community were available. Patients seen by mobile teams were more likely to be detained than those seen in the ED, even after overall risk was controlled for. This finding is in contrast to most studies of mobile crisis services.

Currently, many psychiatric emergency departments offer comprehensive diagnostic services extending well beyond brief screening. Proper diagnosis is important for several reasons, including appropriate disposition. Khuri and Wood (1984) noted a particularly strong association between diagnosis and disposition in an inner-city hospital serving a largely indigent population. The authors noted that a detailed psychosocial and psychiatric history was taken from all patients presenting to this PES. Diagnoses were made according to DSM-III guidelines, and several notable trends emerged. Patients diagnosed with mania or schizophrenia were frequently hospitalized, and patients diagnosed with depression showed a marginally significant trend in this direction. Outpatient treatment was the disposition of choice for patients with substance abuse disorders and adjustment disorders.

Diagnostic accuracy is also important for initiating proper treatment in the the PES. Allen (1996) described a treatment model of the PES that requires specific diagnosis and encourages initiation of treatment. Robins et al. (1977) and Warner and Peabody (1995) indicated that accurate diagnoses can be formulated in the PES, provided that a structured assessment is used. Deferring diagnosis and treatment further delays care unnecessarily. Moreover, the lack of a definitive diagnosis in the PES may lead patients to believe that their time was wasted, causing dissatisfaction and impeding treatment (Allen 1996). An effective PES incorporates elements of triage, psychosocial assessment, and diagnostic evaluation.

Reliability of Psychiatric Assessment in Emergency Settings

Although diagnostic assessment in the PES helps determine disposition, the reliability of diagnosis in routine practice is suspect. In many cases, diagnoses are thought to be inconsistent from one PES to another or between clinicians at the same hospital. Robins et al. (1977) examined the validity of diagnoses made in the PES in blinded reassessments an average of 18.2 months after the initial assessment. Among the 299 patients involved in the study whose cases could be reassessed, the second psychiatrist rater agreed with the initial diagnosis in 84% of cases. This rate of agreement is particularly impressive because many patients had multiple diagnoses and an error in even one would have led the patient to be classified as receiving the wrong diagnosis. Kappa coefficients were consistently above 0.6 for all diagnostic categories, and agreement was significantly better for the most relevant diagnostic categories.

However, Way et al. (1998) examined interrater reliability among psychiatrists in a PES by giving eight experienced emergency psychiatrists videotapes of 30 unstructured, routine PES assessment interviews conducted by psychiatrists. The reviewers were instructed to rate each tape on several patient characteristics, including danger to self, danger to others, psychopathology, depression, psychosis, impulse-control problems, substance abuse, social support, ability to care for self, benefit of inpatient treatment, and patient cooperation. Certain categories (e.g., psychosis and substance abuse) showed high interrater reliability. However, the reviewers' judgments on psychopathology, impulse-control problems, danger to self, and disposition were less consistent with those of the assessing psychiatrist. A dichotomized scale was developed to assess level of agreement among physicians for the diagnosis of patients. In this study of actual interviews, as opposed to Robins et al.'s (1977) earlier work, physicians' assessments matched only 55.5% of the time, as measured by Cohen's kappa—only a 16% improvement over chance.

Warner and Peabody (1995) conducted a retrospective chart review to examine the reliability of diagnoses made by PES residents. For 190 patients, the diagnoses made in the ED were compared with those reported at discharge from an inpatient unit. There proved to be strong agreement for Axis I diagnoses in four major categories: major depression, psychotic-spectrum disorders, bipolar disorders, and substance abuse and dependence disorders. Kappa values of interrater reliability ranged from 0.64 for major depression to 0.87 for substance abuse and dependence disorders.

Taken together, these studies suggest that reliable diagnosis is attainable if that is the focus of the service.

Triage

At triage a rapid initial assessment is made of various aspects of a patient's current clinical status to identify the most acute needs and to direct the patient to the most appropriate initial care. The ED nurse performing triage must simultaneously consider many factors that could potentially be contributing to the patient's presenting condition. An initial assessment of the presenting problem should include observing the patient's behavior, speaking with the patient and collateral contacts, and checking vital signs. The seriousness of the patient's problem should be gauged in terms of risk of self-inflicted injuries, perceived danger to others, and risk of escape from emergency services. The possibility of an acute medical problem requiring immediate attention should also be considered. Ultimately, the triage nurse must determine what measures must be initiated immediately. This may include providing further evaluation promptly, establishing a safe setting for the patient, and determining whether emergency medical attention is required (Dreyfus 1987).

Dreyfus (1987) provided a useful checklist that outlined important considerations for triage nurses (a modified version is presented in Table 2–3). Various scales have been devised to improve the efficiency and consistency of this initial evaluation. Smart et al. (1999) developed a four-tiered Mental Health Triage Scale (MHTS), designed in accordance with the National Triage Scale (NTS), for patients with mental health problems presenting to EDs. The categories, ranging from 2 to 5, represent a continuum of presenting symptom severity and priority of treatment. Category 2 is reserved for emergent care that must occur within 10 minutes of presentation. This applies to patients who present with imminently violent, aggressive, or suicidal behavior. Category 3 refers to patients judged to be in urgent need of care, who are to be seen within 30 minutes. This designation is applied to very distressed or psychotic patients, those likely to deteriorate, those in a situational crisis, or those who are a danger to themselves or others. Category 4 is applied to patients with a long-standing semi-urgent disorder, and category 5 refers to patients with a long-standing nonacute mental health concern.

Although the MHTS does not include an explicit category 1, patients who presented with a life-threatening illness were assigned to category 1 as per the NTS. These patients received immediate medical treatment. Thorough physical examinations were given to patients in categories 2 and 3 prior to consultation with liaison psychiatry. Those in categories 4 and 5 were referred to a liaison psychiatry team after an emergency mental health assessment and appropriate physical examination. The MHTS proved to be a valuable tool for triage, associated with decreases in waiting and transit times and reduction in the number of patients who left without evaluation (Smart et al. 1999).

Bengelsdorf et al. (1984) developed the Crisis Triage Rating Scale (CTRS) to structure the screening of patients presenting to PESs. This measure consisted of a Likert-type rating scale, which required a rating of 1 to 5 on three measures thought to be predic-

Table 2–3. Triage checklist for patients presenting to an emergency department with psychiatric problems

Identifying problems
Observe the patient's behavior.
Have the patient describe presenting problem.
Gather data from collateral contacts.
Check vital signs.
Look for indications of physical illness.
Check current medications.
Ascertain medical and psychiatric histories.

Assessing seriousness of problem
Determine whether the patient is a risk to self or others.
Determine whether the patient presents an escape risk.
Consider whether the patient's symptoms may be due to a medical problem.

Immediate nursing care measures
Assess how long the patient can wait for further evaluation.
Prepare the environment for the patient to wait safely (e.g., remove potentially dangerous objects).
Determine what measures are needed to prevent an immediate medical emergency.

Source. Based on Dreyfus 1987.

tive of disposition decision. Factors included the degree of the patient's dangerousness to self or others, the capability and willingness of the patient's family or support network to assist in treatment, and the patient's motivation and ability to comply with outpatient treatment. A preliminary assessment of this measure indicated that CTRS correctly predicted disposition in 291 (97%) of 300 cases. A score of 8 or lower on the CTRS was thought to be indicative of the need for admission. In a follow-up validation study, 122 psychiatric patients were followed for a 6-month period. Among the 35 patients with scores of 3 to 8, 32 (91%) were ultimately admitted (Bengelsdorf et al. 1984).

To determine the actual validity of the CTRS, Turner and Turner (1991) replicated part of the research done on the CTRS with a sample of 500 emergency psychiatric patients seen at a

London teaching hospital. When a cut-off score of 8 was used as an indicator of admission, CTRS scores were found to be concordant with clinical disposition in 313 (62.2%) of 500 cases, a rate significantly lower than that found in the initial study. However, Turner and Turner found that raising the cut-off score for admission to 9 and to 10 increased concordance to 75.2% and to 81.2%, respectively. They ultimately recommended a cut-off score of 9 for clinical use (Turner and Turner 1991).

Legal Considerations at Triage

Triage is a critical juncture in emergency evaluation, since at that time it is determined how assessment and treatment will proceed. In addition to the many clinical factors that determine how a patient will be referred, there are significant legal considerations. Many of the legal concerns related to emergency medicine center on the Emergency Medical Treatment and Active Labor Act (EMTALA). EMTALA requires that any hospital that participates in Medicare and Medicaid provide medical screening to any patient who is in active labor or seeking emergency care (Weiss and Martinez 1999). If this screening reveals an emergency medical condition, serious threat to life, or active labor, the hospital must provide stabilizing treatment to the extent of its capabilities (Lee 2000). EMTALA defines an emergency medical condition as severe acute symptoms that could reasonably be expected to result in complications in the absence of medical attention (Weiss and Martinez 1999). This definition also applies to acute psychiatric symptoms. Congress passed this legislation in 1986 to prevent the inappropriate transfer of patients who were unable to pay for their care (Diekema 1995). Hospitals may transfer patients in emergency situations only if they lack the resources to treat and only if the benefits outweigh the risks (Lee 2000).

The obligations implied by EMTALA extend beyond emergency services, in that an emergency medical condition that arises on an inpatient unit must be addressed in the same manner. An individual who suffers physical harm as a result of a participating hospital's violation of EMTALA may initiate legal proceedings against the hospital and obtain damages under federal law (Weiss and Martinez 1999). Moreover, a hospital or physician who negligently violates EMTALA may be fined up to $50,000, irrespective of any harm done to the patient (Diekema 1995). Consequently, when an individual presents to triage, it is particularly important to accurately assess the seriousness of physical and psychiatric symptoms for legal as well as medical reasons. Certainly, an assessment of the risk of self-harm must be accomplished. Table 2–4 suggests one approach to this issue.

Table 2–4. Suicide risk assessment guidelines: Thienhaus's recommendations for assessing suicide risk

---

Determine the severity of the patient's stressors and suicide precipitants.

Establish where the patient is on a continuum of suicidality.

Identify accompanying psychopathology and associated risks.

Assess how realistic the patient's plan is.

Outline the patient's personal deterrents to committing suicide.

Recognize the limited benefit of labeling a patient's behavior as manipulative.

Consider the situation awaiting the patient after discharge.

If unsure of level of risk, request a second opinion.

Do not discharge an intoxicated patient.

Document disposition and its rationale.

Source. Adapted from Thienhaus and Piasecki 1997.

Psychosocial Assessment

If a crisis or emergency exists, it is important to conduct a thorough psychosocial assessment to determine precipitants and exacerbating factors relevant to the presenting psychiatric condition. This involves a multifactorial assessment of the patient's functioning and environment (Table 2–5). This assessment should explore the nature and availability of the patient's support system as well as the patient's capacity to use it. Both the extent of the patient's personal danger and his or her dangerousness to others should be assessed. The patient's psychiatric history and current psychiatric status should both be ascertained to determine the patient's present functioning relative to baseline. It is also important to examine the patient's previous methods of coping with similar psychological stressors in the past. The patient's ability to perform basic self-care measures and his or her capacity to participate in treatment also have a significant bearing on the recommended course of therapy. Finally, the requests of the patient and the patient's family should be considered in determining a disposition (Gerson and Bassuk 1980). Treatment would appear to have a greater likelihood of success if it has the approval of the patient and the patient's family.

Table 2–5. Information to ascertain in a psychosocial evaluation

Availability of a support system and the patient's capacity to use it
Dangerousness of a patient to self and others
Psychiatric history and current psychiatric status
Patient's previous methods of coping with similar stressors
Ability to conduct self-care measures
Motivation and capacity to participate in the treatment process
Requests of patients and family

Source. Based on Gerson and Bassuk 1980.

More recently, additional measures have been suggested as adjuncts to the standard psychosocial assessment. Currier and Briere (2000), noting the high prevalence of domestic and interpersonal violence in those receiving care in the PES, suggested that it might be useful to employ a screening measure of traumatic violence in the PES assessment. In a prospective analysis, these authors employed a standardized trauma interview measure to evaluate histories of childhood physical abuse, childhood sexual abuse, sexual assault or rape as a child or adolescent, adult sexual assault or rape, adult spouse abuse, and adult nonintimate violence. Among the 167 PES patients interviewed, victimization rates ranged from 10% for victims of peer sexual assault in childhood to 45% for victims of child physical abuse. Since trauma histories are associated with depression, personality disorders, and substance abuse, high victimization rates displayed among these PES patients indicated that it may be worthwhile to incorporate a measure of trauma into the psychosocial assessment.

Diagnostic Assessment

Although current practice in the PES requires some level of diagnostic assessment, the appropriate level of evaluation has not been established. Even prior to DSM-III-R, Lieberman and Baker (1985) found a reasonable level of reliability for broad diagnostic categories, including psychosis, depression, and alcoholism. These authors felt that recognition of general diagnostic categories was sufficient for initiation of treatment in an emergency and that diagnosis could be completed in an inpatient or outpatient setting if timely access to those services is available.

Personnel

Perhaps the most important aspect of assessment in emergency psychiatry is the qualifications of the personnel performing the evaluations. A multidisciplinary team led by a psychiatrist is ideal. Psychiatrists are able to provide expert consultation in the differential diagnosis of thought and mood disorders. However, many psychiatric EDs, particularly those that do not offer comprehensive services, cannot provide continuous coverage by a psychiatrist (Allen 1999; Slaby 1981). As a result, psychiatric nurses, social workers, and less frequently, psychologists can intervene with crisis intervention and brief psychotherapy. Commonly, psychiatric nurses and social workers perform initial data collection and assessment prior to calling in a psychiatrist for diagnostic assessment (Slaby 1981). Presumably, nurses have the advantage of being trained to detect medical causes of behavioral emergencies.

Currently, the standards for emergency psychiatric assessment vary significantly between states and individual institutions. PESs minimally provide screening and referral to patients presenting with acute psychiatric complaints. Level 1 services provide a more comprehensive diagnostic assessment, with the objective of rapidly initiating therapy. In emergency settings in which psychiatrists are not readily available, diagnostic assessment may need to be deferred and treatment focused on crisis stabilization and referral.

Cognitive Screening in the PES

A cognitive screen is a brief performance-based assessment that measures one or more domains of cognitive function (Anastasi and Urbina 1997; Mitrushina and Fuld 1996). Cognitive screening may enhance the diagnostic process, facilitating appropriate treatment strategies and use of psychiatric services, such as reducing unnecessary hospitalization (Gold et al. 1999; Hobart et al. 1999; Mitrushina and Fuld 1996; Spitzer et al. 1999; Zimmerman and Mattia 1999). Perhaps the most widely used cognitive screening measure in the PES is the Mini-Mental State Exam (MMSE; Folstein et al. 1975). The MMSE was originally designed to assess change in cognitive impairment in geriatric inpatients. Over the years, the MMSE has come to be used routinely as the cognitive screening instrument in the PES. The instrument has gained popularity because it is easy to administer and assesses a wide range of cognitive functions in verbal and some visual modalities. A factor-analytic study, for example, found that the MMSE tapped frontal, memory, and spatial domains of cognitive functioning in psychiatric patients (de Leon et al. 1998). The MMSE also identifies individuals with a high probability of moderate to severe global cognitive impairment, especially in elderly patients presenting for treatment (Dziedzic et al. 1998).

The MMSE, however, has important limitations (Bowie et al. 1999; Folstein 1998; Lamarre and Patten 1991). Although it is an excellent screening device for detecting severe dementias, it has inadequate sensitivity for detecting milder forms of dementia and cognitive dysfunction in elderly patients and psychiatric patients (Faustman et al. 1990; Nuechterlein and Subotnik 1996; Wind et al. 1997). Underdetection of cognitive impairment in patients presenting for emergency psychiatric treatment may result in inappropriate PES triage decisions.

Along with the MMSE, clinician-based ratings of cognitive deficits (e.g., symptom ratings of disorientation, loss of abstract reasoning, and concentration impairment) are also routinely used in the PES to assess cognitive impairment. A recent study, however, found that symptom-based ratings of various types of cognitive dysfunction lack convergent validity with performance-based measures of the same constructs (Harvey et al., in press). A clinical rating of "poor attention span" is measuring something different from a performance-based measure of poor attention and may not adequately measure the full extent of a patient's cognitive impairment or its functional consequences.

As a result, the use of performance-based cognitive screening examinations in the PES is needed. Cognitive screens may help PES clinicians detect disorders that are commonly missed by the standard intake psychiatric interview. For example, patients presenting with comorbid substance abuse, violent patients, and patients experiencing mild disorientation are particularly prone to underdetection during routine psychiatric examination (Marson et al. 1988; McNiel et al. 1992; Rabinowitz and Garelik-Wyler 1999; Wilkins et al. 1991). Use of cognitive screens, moreover, may enhance PES diagnostic and treatment decisions while minimizing the time, resources, and cost of service delivery to patients presenting for emergency services (Wind et al. 1997).

Screens can measure various domains of cognitive dysfunction that may characterize particular groups of patients. The cognitive screens described below are illustrative (and by no means exhaustive) of appropriate measures of cognitive functioning in PES assessment.

Trailmaking Test

The Trialmaking Test (TMT) is a particularly useful cognitive screen because of its accessibility, ease of use, and modifiability. The TMT is given in two parts (Part A and B). Part A requires the patient to draw lines to consecutively numbered circles on a worksheet. Part B requires concentration and cognitive flexibility skills as patients must shift sets by drawing lines connecting numbered to lettered circles (e.g., 1, to A, to 2, to B, etc.). This format has been modified for use with non–English speaking populations, using two colors (pink and yellow) rather than letters. In the Color Trails, Part A remains essentially the same as in the TMT, but Part B requires the patient to match numbers with colors in a progressive and alternating pattern (i.e., 1 yellow, 1 pink, 2 yellow, 2 pink, etc.).

Combining the TMT with the Visual Reproduction subtest of the Wechsler Memory Scale (WMS; Wechsler 1981) has shown great clinical utility in evaluating various groups of subjects (Galynker and Harvey 1992; Gfeller et al. 1995). The WMS Visual Reproduction requires the patient to copy four designs following a brief presentation (10 seconds each) and again approximately 30 minutes later. Use of this combined screen was found to successfully discriminate among patients presenting to the PES with schizophrenia, mood disorder, or adjustment disorder (Galynker and Harvey 1992). The screen was also able to detect increased levels of cognitive impairment in patients with schizophrenia or mood disorders relative to patients with adjustment disorder. Poor performance on this screen in the PES, moreover, predicted increased likelihood of admission to the hospital (Galynker and Harvey 1992).

California Verbal Learning Test

The California Verbal Learning Test (CVLT; Delis et al. 1987) has also been used successfully in the PES to differentiate psychiatric conditions. The CVLT measures patients' verbal learning and memory ability. Sixteen words are presented to the patient, who is then instructed to repeat them back. Following a delay period, the patient is then asked to recall the words again, providing a measure of long-term recall. The test also has both recall and recognition conditions. A recent study found that CVLT performance profiles discriminated among cocaine abusers, schizophrenic patients, and cocaine-abusing schizophrenic patients presenting to the PES (Serper et al. 2000a, 2000b). Group patterns of CVLT deficits, moreover, were better at discriminating between diagnostic groups than clinical assessment ratings of presenting symptoms (Serper et al. 1999). It was found that cocaine-abusing schizophrenic patients presented a CVLT profile marked by severe forgetting of previously acquired CVLT information, compared with the other groups, who retained acquired information. In contrast, tests of sustained attention, distractibility, abstract reasoning, and executive functioning did not discriminate between groups (Serper et al. 2000b). These results, if confirmed by future studies, suggest that cocaine-abusing schizophrenic patients present to the PES with severe cognitive deficits marked by forgetting of recently acquired information. This is an important issue, because very large subgroups of psychiatric patients meet diagnostic criteria for substance abuse or dependence. Consequently, a potentially significant source of clinical and cognitive dysfunction often may remain unrecognized and untreated during an acute psychiatric admission.

Additionally, the CVLT, unlike the MMSE, may also be useful in the PES because it can aid clinicians in differentiating patients with a cortical from subcortical dementia (Delis et al. 1991; Peavy et al. 1994; Roman et al. 1998). Although there is heterogeneity of cognitive dysfunction among patients with various types of subcortical dementias (Roman et al. 1998), patients presenting with subcortical dementias such as symptomatic HIV, Huntington's disease, or Parkinson's disease manifest a similar pattern of generalized retrieval deficits on verbal memory tasks (Bondi et al. 1996; Delis et al. 1991; Peavy et al. 1994; Roman et al. 1998). In contrast to patients with subcortical dementia, patients with Alzheimer's disease show recognition deficits, semantic knowledge deficits, and deficits in their ability to acquire new information. For example, on the CVLT, Alzheimer's patients fail to show a normal improvement in performance when recognition memory is tested rather than recall memory (Delis et al. 1991). Patients with Huntington's disease, in contrast, identify more target items during recognition testing than during free recall trials (Roman et al. 1998). Alzheimer's patients also demonstrate significantly more intrusion errors than Huntington's, symptomatic HIV-positive, and Parkinson's patients.

One important drawback to using the CVLT as a PES cognitive screen is that it is laborious to administer. It can take 40–60 minutes to complete and requires patient cooperation and sustained attention. An alternative may be to use a less taxing assessment of verbal learning and memory like the Rey Auditory-Verbal Learning Test (RAVLT). The RAVLT also requires serial learning of word lists, which may prove to be a more facile cognitive screen than the more comprehensive CVLT but may still be sensitive enough to help the PES clinician formulate diagnoses and make treatment decisions. As mentioned earlier, however, complex screens have been successfully administered to acute patients in the PES, so more lengthy screens, like the CVLT, should not be excluded outright.

Clock Drawing Test

Research investigating the use of other cognitive screens has led to advances in early detection of Alzheimer's disease, in tracking dementia progression, and in assessing the efficacy of potential therapeutic drugs (Bondi et al. 1996; Savage 1997). With Alzheimer's disease constituting the most common cause of dementia (with estimates indicating that it affects approximately 4 million people in the United States [Khachturian et al. 1994]) and frequent PES visitation (Coyne and Gjertsen 1993; Lagomasino et al. 1999), cognitive screening may be particularly useful in differentiating behavioral symptoms caused by psychiatric conditions from symptoms caused by an underlying dementia. The Clock Drawing Test (CDT) shows great promise as a PES screen for Alzheimer's disease because it is easy to administer and is sensitive to detecting cognitive disturbances associated with that disease (Tracy et al. 1996).

Although slightly different scoring procedures exist for the CDT, Lezak (1995) provides the criteria for evaluating drawings on a 10-point scale, with 10 points representing a well-executed drawing (e.g., the clock hands in approximately correct position) and 1 point indicating a noninterpretable outcome or no attempt at all. Research using the CDT indicates that patients with Alzheimer's disease demonstrate deficiencies on this task relative to schizophrenic patients and patients with other types of dementias (Wolf-Klein et al. 1989). It was found in clinical settings outside the PES, for example, that over 94% of those with probable Alzheimer's disease scored in the impaired range on the CDT, compared with 60% of patients with other types of dementia and 22% of patients with functional psychosis (Tracy et al. 1996; Wolf-Klein et al. 1989). CDT deficits in patients with Alzheimer's disease also appear to increase over time, resulting in a steady decline in CDT global performance (Savage 1997). As opposed to the deteriorating course observed in Alzheimer's patients, CDT global performance in schizophrenic patients does not vary with the duration or chronicity of their illness (Lezak 1995).

Additionally, patients with Alzheimer's disease have been distinguished from other groups by the types of errors they make on the CDT. Interestingly, the pattern of CDT errors committed by Alzheimer's patients involves conceptual deficits (i.e., difficulty in the production of a clock face). Patients with various types of subcortical dementias and those with vascular dementias, in contrast, produce a relatively greater number of CDT spatial or planning deficits (i.e., gaps in clock numbers or other disorganization of layout) (Wolf-Klein et al. 1989). These planning problems are not weighted heavily in the global performance measure and likely account for the lower proportion of impaired range scores seen in other groups. In addition, the conceptual errors Alzheimer's patients make appear to occur early in the illness course (Bondi et al. 1996), suggesting that the use of the CDT in the PES may be a particularly sensitive screen for Alzheimer's disease detection. These studies strongly suggest that the CDT provides useful information in discriminating between Alzheimer's disease and functional psychoses and other types of dementias. Unlike the CVLT, however, CDT global performance scores were poor at discriminating substance-abusing schizophrenic patients from their nonabusing counterparts (Tracy et al. 1996).

Cognitive screens hold the promise of improving psychiatric service delivery by increasing sensitivity to detection of impairment that may be missed during the traditional PES interview or mental status examination. Cognitive screens, in addition, may offer an important time-saving function during determination of patient disposition because they can help clarify the extent of functional impairment. While the broad appeal of the MMSE comes from its wide-ranging assessment, the MMSE is not sensitive to detection of cognitive deficits in many groups of psychiatric and dementia patients. PES clinicians should incorporate additional cognitive screening instruments when they are attempting to make differential diagnoses and when disposition decisions are unclear.

References

Allen MH: Definitive treatment in the psychiatric emergency service. Psychiatr Q 67:247–262, 1996

Allen MH: Level 1 psychiatric emergency services: the tools of the crisis sector. Psychiatr Clin North Am 22:713–734, 1999

American College of Emergency Physicians: Clinical policy for the initial approach to patients presenting with altered mental status. Ann Emerg Med 33:251–281, 1999

Anastasi A, Urbina S: Psychological Testing, 7th Edition. Upper Saddle River, NJ, Prentice-Hall, 1997

Bengelsdorf H, Levy LE, Emerson RL, et al: A crisis triage rating scale: brief dispositional assessment of patients at risk for hospitalization. J Nerv Ment Dis 172:424–430, 1984

Bondi MW, Salmon DP, Kasniak AW: The neuropsychology of dementia, in Neuropsychological Assessment of Neuropsychiatric Disorders, 2nd Edition. Edited by Grant I, Adams KM. New York, Oxford University Press, 1996, pp 164–199

Bowie P, Branton T, Holmes J: Should the Mini Mental State Examination be used to monitor dementia treatments? Lancet 354(9189):1527–1528, 1999

Brown EJ, Jemmott LS: HIV among people with mental illness: contributing factors, prevention needs, barriers, and strategies. Journal of Psychosocial Nursing 38:14–19, 2000

Carlson RJ, Nayar N, Suh M: Physical disorders among emergency psychiatric patients. Can J Psychiatry 26:65–67, 1981

Carney CP, Yates WR, Goerdt CJ, et al: Psychiatrists' and internists' knowledge and attitudes about delivery of clinical preventive medical services. Psychiatr Serv 49:1594–1600, 1998

Coyne AC, Gjertsen R: Characteristics of older adults referred to a psychiatric emergency outreach service. J Ment Health Admin 20:208–211, 1993

Currier GW, Briere J: Trauma orientation and detection of violence histories in the psychiatric emergency service. J Nerv Ment Dis 188:622–624, 2000

de Leon J, Baca-Garcia E, Simpson GM: A factor analysis of the Mini-Mental State Examination in schizophrenic disorders. Acta Psychiatr Scand 98:366–368, 1998

Delis DC, Kramer JH, Kaplan E, et al: California Verbal Learning Test. San Antonio, TX, Psychological Corporation, 1987

Delis DC, Massman PJ, Butters N: Profiles of demented and amnesic patients on the California Verbal Learning Test: implications for the assessment of memory disorders. Psychol Assess 3:19–26, 1991

Diekema DS: Unwinding the COBRA: new perspectives on EMTALA. Pediatr Emerg Care 11:243–248, 1995

Dreyfus JK: Nursing assessment of the ED patient with psychiatric symptoms: a quick reference. J Emerg Nurs 13:278–282, 1987

Dziedzic L, Brady WJ, Lindsay R, et al: The use of the Mini-Mental Status Examination in the ED evaluation of the elderly. Am J Emerg Med 16:686–689, 1998

Engleman NB, Jobes DA, Berman AL, et al: Clinicians' decision making about involuntary commitment. Psychiatr Serv 49:941–945, 1998

Faustman WO, Moses JA, Csernansky JG: Limitations of the Mini-Mental State Examination in predicting neuropsychological functioning in a psychiatric sample. Acta Psychiatr Scand 81:126–131, 1990

Folstein MF: Mini-Mental and son. Int J Geriatr Psychiatry 13:290–294, 1998

Folstein MF, Folstein SE, McHugh PR: "Mini-Mental State'": a practical method for grading the cognitive state of patients for the clinician. J Psychiatr Res 12:189–198, 1975

Galynker II, Harvey PD: Neuropsychological screening in the psychiatric emergency room. Compr Psychiatry 33:291–295, 1992

Gerson S, Bassuk E: Psychiatric emergencies: an overview. Am J Psychiatry 137:1–11, 1980

Gfeller JD, Meldrum DL, Jacobi A: The impact of constructional impairment on the WMS-R Visual Reproduction subtests. J Clin Psychol 51: 58–63, 1995

Gold JM, Queern C, Iannone VN, et al: Repeatable battery for the assessment of neuropsychological status as a screening test in schizophrenia, I: sensitivity, reliability, and validity. Am J Psychiatry 156:1944–1950, 1999

Golomb BA, Pyne JM, Wright B, et al: The role of psychiatrists in primary care of patients with severe mental illness. Psychiatr Serv 51:766–773, 2000

Hall R, Popkin MK, Devaul RA, et al: Physical illness presenting as psychiatric disease. Arch Gen Psychiatry 35:1315–1320, 1978

Hall R, Gardner ER, Popkin MK, et al: Unrecognized physical illness prompting psychiatric admission: a prospective study. Am J Psychiatry 138:629–635, 1981

Harvey PD, Serper MR, White L, et al: Convergent validity of cognitive symptom and cognitive performance measures. Compr Psychiatry (in press)

Hatta K, Takahashi T, Nakamura H, et al: Abnormal physiological conditions in acute schizophrenic patients on emergency admission: dehydration, hypokalemia, leukocytosis, and elevated serum muscle enzymes. Eur Arch Psychiatry Clin Neurosci 248:180–188, 1998

Henneman PL, Mendoza R, Lewis RJ: Prospective evaluation of emergency department medical clearance. Ann Emerg Med 24:672–677, 1994

Hobart MP, Goldberg R, Bartko JJ, et al: Repeatable battery for the assessment of neuropsychological status as a screening test in schizophrenia, II: convergent/discriminant validity and diagnostic group comparisons. Am J Psychiatry 156:1951–1957, 1999

Hollister LE: Electrocardiographic screening in psychiatric patients. J Clin Psychiatry 65:26–29, 1995

Jacobs D: Evaluation and management of the violent patient in emergency settings. Psychiatr Clin North Am 6:259–269, 1983

Karasu TB, Waltzman SA, Lindenmayer JP, et al: The medical care of patients with psychiatric illness. Hosp Community Psychiatry 31: 463–472, 1980

Kaufman DM, Zun L: A quantifiable, brief mental status examination for emergency patients. J Emerg Med 13:449–456, 1995

Khachturian ZS, Phelps CH, Buckholtz NS: The prospect of developing treatments for Alzheimer disease, in Alzheimer Disease. Edited by Terry RD, Katzman KL, Bick M. New York, Raven, 1994, pp 445–454

Khuri R, Wood K: The role of diagnosis in a psychiatric emergency setting. Hosp Community Psychiatry 35:715–718, 1984

Kick SD, Morrison M, Kathol RG: Medical training in psychiatry residency: a proposed curriculum. Gen Hospital Psychiatry 19:259–266, 1997

Knutsen E, DuRand C: Previously unrecognized physical illnesses in psychiatric patients. Hosp Community Psychiatry 42:182–186, 1991

Koran LM, Sox HC, Marton KI, et al: Medical evaluation of psychiatric patients. Arch Gen Psychiatry 46:733–740, 1989

Koranyi EK: Somatic illness in psychiatric patients. Psychosomatics 21: 887–891, 1980

Korn CS, Currier GW, Henderson SO: "Medical clearance" of psychiatric patients without medical complaints in the emergency department. J Emerg Med 18:173–176, 2000

Lamarre CJ, Patten SB: Evaluation of the Modified Mini-Mental State Examination in a general psychiatric population. Can J Psychiatry 36: 507–511, 1991

Lagomasino I, Daly R, Stoudemire A: Medical assessment of patients presenting with psychiatric symptoms in the emergency setting. Psychiatr Clin North Am 22:819–850, 1999

Lee NG: Update on EMTALA. Am J Nurs 100:57–58, 2000

Lezak MD: Neuropsychological Assessment, 3rd Edition. New York, Oxford University Press, 1995

Lieberman AA, Coburn AF: The health of the chronically mentally ill: a review of the literature. Community Ment Health J 22:104–116, 1986

Lieberman PB, Baker FM: The reliability of psychiatric diagnosis in the emergency room. Hosp Community Psychiatry 36:291–293, 1985

Lima BR, Pai S: Concurrent medical and psychiatric disorders among schizophrenic and neurotic outpatients. Community Ment Health J 23:30–39, 1987

Marson DC, McGovern MP, Pomp HC: Psychiatric decision making in the psychiatric emergency room: a research overview. Am J Psychiatry 145:918–925, 1988

McNiel DE, Myers RS, Zeiner HK, et al: The role of violence in decisions about hospitalization from the psychiatric emergency room. Am J Psychiatry 149:207–212, 1992

Mitrushina M, Fuld PA: Cognitive screening methods, in Neuropsychological Assessment of Neuropsychiatric Disorders, 2nd Edition. Edited by Grant I, Adams KM. New York, Oxford University Press; 1996, pp 118–138

Nuechterlein KH, Subotnik KL: The role of neurocognitive deficits in understanding adaptive functioning in severe psychiatric illness: commentary on Hawkins and Cooper. Psychiatry 59:389–392, 1996

Olshaker JS, Browne B, Jerrard DA, et al: Medical screening and clearance of psychiatric patients in the emergency department. Acad Emerg Med 4:124–128, 1997

Peavy G, Jacobs D, Salmon DP, et al: Verbal memory performance of patients with human immunodeficiency virus infection: evidence of subcortical dysfunction. The HNRC Group. J Clin Exp Neuropsychol 16:508–523, 1994

Rabinowitz J, Garelik-Wyler R: Accuracy and confidence in clinical assessment of psychiatric inpatients risk of violence. Int J Law Psychiatry 22:99–106, 1999

Rabinowitz J, Massad A, Fennig S: Factors influencing disposition decisions for patients seen in a psychiatric emergency service. Psychiatr Serv 46:712–718, 1995

Riba M, Hale M: Medical clearance: fact or fiction in the hospital emergency room. Psychosomatics 31:400–404, 1990

Robins E, Gentry KA, Munoz RA, et al: A contrast of the three more common illnesses with the ten less common in a study and 18-month follow-up of 314 psychiatric emergency room patients. Arch Gen Psychiatry 34:285–291, 1977

Roman MJ, Delis DC, Filoteo JV, et al: Is there a "subcortical" profile of attentional dysfunction? A comparison of patients with Huntington's and Parkinson's diseases on a global-local focused attention tasks. J Clin Exp Neuropsychol 20:873–874, 1998

Savage CR: Neuropsychology of subcortical dementias. Psychiatr Clin North Am 20:911–931, 1997

Schuster JM, Thienhaus OJ, Ventura M: Usefulness of physical examinations in the psychiatric emergency service. Psychiatr Serv 47:575–576, 1996

Segal SP, Watson MA, Goldfinger SM, et al: Civil commitment in the psychiatric emergency room, I: the assessment of dangerousness by emergency room clinicians. Arch Gen Psychiatry 45:748–752, 1988a

Segal SP, Watson MA, Goldfinger SM, et al: Civil commitment in the emergency room, II: mental disorder indicators and three dangerousness criteria. Arch Gen Psychiatry 45:753–758, 1988b

Segal SP, Watson MA, Goldfinger SM, et al: Civil commitment in the psychiatric emergency room, III: disposition as a function of mental disorder and dangerousness indicators. Arch Gen Psychiatry 45:759–763, 1988c

Segal SP, Laurie TA, Segal MJ: Factors in the use of coercive retention in civil commitment evaluations in psychiatric emergency services. Psychiatr Serv 52:514–520, 2001

Serper MR, Chou JC, Allen MH, et al: Symptomatic overlap of cocaine intoxication and acute schizophrenia at emergency presentation. Schizophr Bull 25:387–394, 1999

Serper MR, Bergman A, Copersino ML, et al: Learning and memory impairment in cocaine-dependent and comorbid schizophrenic patients. Psychiatry Res 93:21–32, 2000a

Serper MR, Copersino ML, Richarme D, et al: Neurocognitive functioning in recently abstinent, cocaine-abusing schizophrenic patients. J Subst Abuse 11:205–213, 2000b

Slaby AE: Emergency psychiatry in the general hospital: staffing, training, and leadership issues. Gen Hospital Psychiatry 3:306–309, 1981

Smart D, Pollard C, Walpole B: Mental health triage in emergency medicine. Aust N Z J Psychiatry 33:57–66, 1999

Sox HC, Koran LM, Sox CH, et al: A medical algorithm for detecting physical disease in psychiatric patients. Hosp Community Psychiatry 12:1270–1276, 1989

Spitzer RL, Kroenke K, Williams JB: Validation and utility of a self-report version of PRIME-MD: the PHQ Primary Care Study. Primary Care Evaluation of Mental Disorders. Patient Health Questionnaire. JAMA 282:1737–1744, 1999

Summers WK, Munoz RA, Read MR: The psychiatric physical examination, Part I: methodology. J Clin Psychiatry 42:95–98, 1981a

Summers WK, Munoz RA, Read WR, et al: The psychiatric physical examination, Part II: findings in 75 unselected psychiatric patients. J Clin Psychiatry 42:99–102, 1981b

Thienhaus OJ: Rational physical evaluation in the emergency room. Hosp Community Psychiatry 43:311–312, 1992

Thienhaus OJ, Piasecki M: Assessment of suicide risk. Psychiatr Serv 48:293–294, 1997

Tintinalli J, Peacock FW, Wright MA: Emergency medical evaluation of psychiatric patients. Ann Emerg Med 23:859–862, 1994

Tracy JI, deLeon J, Doonan R, et al: Clock drawing in schizophrenia. Psychol Rep 79:923–928, 1996

Turner PM, Turner TJ: Validation of the Crisis Triage Rating Scale for Psychiatric Emergencies. Can J Psychiatry 36:651–654, 1991

Viner MW, Waite J, Thienhaus OJ: Comorbidity and the need for physical examinations among patients seen in the psychiatric emergency service. Psychiatr Serv 47:947–948, 1996

Wallace SR, Ward JT, Goldberg RJ, et al: The social worker as primary psychiatric consultant to the general hospital emergency room. Emergency Health Services Review 3:11–24, 1985

Warner MD, Peabody CA: Reliability of diagnoses made by psychiatric residents in a general emergency department. Psychiatr Serv 46:1284–1286, 1995

Waxman HM, Dubin W, Klein M, et al: Geriatric psychiatry in the emergency department, II: evaluation and treatment of geriatric and nongeriatric admissions. J Am Geriatr Society 32:343–349, 1984

Way BB, Banks S: Clinical factors related to admission and release decisions in psychiatric emergency services. Psychiatr Serv 52:214–218, 2001

Way BB, Allen MH, Mumpower JL, et al: Interrater agreement among psychiatrists in psychiatric emergency assessments. Am J Psychiatry 155:1423–1428, 1998

Wechsler D: Wechsler Memory Scale. New York, Psychological Corporation, 1981

Weiss LD, Martinez JA: Fixing EMTALA: what's wrong with the Patient Transfer Act. Journal of Public Health Policy 20:335–347, 1999

Wilkins JN, Shaner AL, Patterson CM, et al: Discrepancies among patient report, clinical assessment, and urine analysis in psychiatric patients during inpatient admission. Psychopharmacol Bull 27:149–154, 1991

Williams ER, Shepherd SM: Medical clearance of psychiatric patients. Emerg Med Clin North Am 18:185–198, 2000

Wind AW, Schellevis FG, Van Staveren G, et al: Limitations of the Mini-Mental State Examination in diagnosing dementia in general practice. Int J Geriatr Psychiatry 12:101–108, 1997

Wolf-Klein GP, Silverstone FA, Levy AP: Screening for Alzheimer's disease by clock drawing. J Am Geriatr Soc 37:730–734, 1989

Zimmerman M, Mattia JI. The reliability and validity of a screening questionnaire for 13 DSM-IV Axis I disorders (the Psychiatric Diagnostic Screening Questionnaire) in psychiatric outpatients. J Clin Psychiatry 10:677–683, 1999

Chapter 3

Assessment and Treatment of Suicidal Patients in an Emergency Setting

Peter L. Forster, M.D.
Linda H. Wu, B.A.

Suicidal ideation, suicide attempts, and the specter of completed suicide form one of the core problems in emergency psychiatry. Suicidal behavior is present in at least one-third of patients seen in the psychiatric emergency service (PES) (Dhossche 2000), and in some ways, the assessment and management of suicidal patients is the prototype of emergency mental health care.

Epidemiology

Suicide is the eighth leading cause of death in the United States, and more than 30,000 people in the United States kill themselves every year (Centers for Disease Control and Prevention [CDC] 2000). For every two victims of homicide in the United States, there are three people who take their own lives (CDC 2000).

Highlighting the seriousness of working with suicidal patients in the emergency setting is a study by Beck et al. (1985), who found that 7% of patients hospitalized for suicidal ideation without a recent attempt committed suicide during a follow-up period of 5 to 10 years. Another study followed patients who had been treated in an emergency room after self-poisoning. At 14-year follow-up, almost 22% of the patients had died and 7% had committed suicide (Suokas 2001).

A recent review of the literature on the epidemiology of suicide attempts found that lifetime prevalence rates ranged from 728 to 5,930 per 100,000 individuals (Welch 2001). Every day, approximately 86 Americans take their own lives and 1,500 make suicide attempts (CDC 2000). Drawing on this and other information that highlights the public health significance of suicide, U.S. Surgeon General David Satcher developed a National Strategy for Suicide Prevention. Key goals of this national strategy (U.S. Public Health Service 1999) include

- Developing and implementing suicide prevention programs.
- Promoting efforts to reduce access to lethal means and methods of self-harm.
- Implementing training for the recognition of at-risk behavior and for the delivery of effective treatment.
- Developing and promoting effective clinical and professional practices.
- Improving access to and community linkages with mental health and substance abuse services.

Many of these goals are relevant to a discussion of suicide in the emergency setting. In this chapter, we particularly highlight the importance of reducing access to lethal means of self-harm, improving access to mental health and substance abuse services, and developing more effective treatment in the emergency service.

The primary focus of this chapter is on a subset of individuals who commit suicide: those who have had some contact with the mental health system prior to their suicide. Considering the population of individuals who commit suicide despite evaluation by a mental health professional, there is evidence of considerable opportunities to improve care. For instance, Malone et al. (1995) found that physicians failed to document a suicide history in one-quarter of patients identified by a research assessment as having made a suicide attempt and as being currently depressed. We discuss the broad spectrum of suicidal ideation and suicide attempts and distinguish it from deliberate repetitive self-aggression. Suicide prevention programs that reach out to individuals at risk without any formal mental health contact are beyond the scope of this discussion.

The Spectrum of Suicidal Behavior

Attempts Versus Completions

A useful way of classifying suicidal behavior is to consider ideation, planning, attempts, and completed suicide. Attempts may be further subdivided into impulsive and premeditated attempts and medically serious and nonserious attempts. The relationship between ideation, various kinds of attempts, and completed suicide is complex. It does not represent a simple hierarchy of increasing severity.

In the National Comorbidity Survey (Kessler et al. 1999), about 14% of the American population reported having thoughts about suicide, 4% had a plan, and 4.6% had made an attempt. The cumulative probabilities were 34% for the transition from ideation to a plan, 72% from a plan to an attempt, and 26% from ideas of suicide to an unplanned attempt. Note that there are many unplanned attempts. Planned and unplanned attempts followed a somewhat different course: 90% of all unplanned and 60% of planned first attempts occurred within 1 year of the onset of ideation. Thus, thoughts about suicide are clearly a significant risk factor for suicide attempts, especially those after the onset of suicidal ideation.

A history of attempt increases the odds of completion more than any other risk factor. However, psychological autopsy data suggest that most individuals who completed suicide had not made a prior attempt, and at least one study of attempters found that only about 10% ultimately die by suicide (Maris et al. 1992). It would appear, then, that certain kinds of ideation and planning are more serious than certain types of suicide attempts.

Medical Seriousness and Impulsivity

Anyone who has practiced in the PES is aware that there are many individuals who make attempts but who, at least in the short run, do not complete suicide. Recent efforts in the field have focused on identifying a group of individuals who have made medically serious suicide attempts, in order to get more information about those who seem to be at highest risk of suicide. For instance, Elliott et al. (1996) found significant differences between those who made medically serious attempts and those who made non–medically serious attempts. The former group had more patients with unipolar depression (34% vs. 20%) and more patients with substance-induced mood disorder (30% vs. 10%). By contrast, more patients making non–medically serious attempts had bipolar depression (19% vs. 6%) and more had borderline personality disorder (22% vs. 34%). Some evidence suggested that those who made non–medically serious attempts were more impulsive. Other studies have also found a significant inverse relationship between impulsivity and lethality of the suicide attempt (Baca-Garcia et al. 2001).

One of the biggest challenges facing the emergency clinician is the way in which suicidal individuals relate to others. It might seem that those who commit suicide and who are in mental health treatment must have not been seen at the time that they felt suicidal. However, Isometsa et al. (1995) found that of the group of individuals who had had contact with a health professional prior to suicide, 41% had had contact within the months prior to suicide, and almost one-fifth of these individuals had seen the clinician on the day of the suicide.

A minority of patients who commit suicide and who have had contact with health professionals appear to have expressed ideation or intention to their therapists (Earle et al. 1994). Far more often, the final consultation is to acquire more medication (Obafunwa and Busuttil 1994). Suicidal ideation and intention are symptoms of desperation, but some who have such thoughts will not readily share them with a health professional. Thus, efforts to provide intensive treatment to those at highest risk cannot simply rely on self-report of suicidal ideation and planning.

Goals of Emergency Assessment

Sensitivity, Specificity, and the Problem of Prediction

In reviewing the literature on suicide, it is important to identify certain common threads. For instance, there is a large literature on risk factors for suicidal behavior. In reviewing this literature, one might conclude that a simple assessment for all possible risk factors for suicide would identify those individuals who will commit suicide. The problem is that suicide remains, at any given point in time, a rare event. Thus, any test that identifies the majority of individuals who complete suicide (i.e., it is sensitive enough to be useful as a screening tool) is very likely to identify a much larger group of people who do not commit suicide (i.e., it will not be adequately specific). One of the best studies to date (Allgulander and Fisher 1990), a prospective study of nearly 9,000 individuals with high suicide risk who were evaluated with a comprehensive clinical battery of assessment tools and statistical analysis, failed to find any clinical predictors that could successfully identify future completers and distinguish that group from the much larger group of individuals who would not complete suicide. Similarly, Pokorny (1983) found that in a sample of 4,800 patients consecutively admitted to an inpatient psychiatric service, there was no set of measures that did not both miss many at-risk cases and erroneously identify too many other individuals as being at risk. The author concluded that identifying individuals who will commit suicide is not currently feasible.

A landmark study by Motto and Bostrom (1990a) suggested that a relatively small number of items could predict individuals who would commit suicide (with a sensitivity of 79%). However, a follow-up study conducted by Motto and Bostrom (1990b) found that these criteria did not predict suicide with a different group of subjects. Thus, to date, every attempt to identify a simple scale or set of scales to distinguish between those who commit suicide and those who do not has failed.

Prediction Versus Treatment

What are the goals of the emergency evaluation of a potentially suicidal individual? From one perspective, the goal is to identify those at greatest risk in order to place them in secure environments and prevent them from acting on their impulses. This is an essentially linear view of the assessment process. Success is measured by the hospitalization of those at highest risk. When we evaluated the factors that distinguished patients who committed suicide after a PES evaluation from the factors that were associated with a high perceived risk but not with suicide, we found that all of the patients who committed suicide within 6 months of a PES visit had been hospitalized (P. L. Forster, ms. in submission). From the "triage" perspective this represents a success, but from a treatment perspective it raises the issue of what other steps might have been taken to prevent suicide. One issue that we touch on later is that suicide seems to be associated with disrupted treatment relationships and that in many systems there is often poor continuity of care from inpatient to outpatient treatment.

It is our contention that the goals of emergency evaluation are different than simply a triage assessment. Suicidal ideation and suicide attempts must be thought of as potentially severe symptoms of psychiatric illness, and the focus of assessment should be on finding the best treatment for that illness. This "treatment" perspective suggests that taking a risk (deciding not to hospitalize a patient because outpatient treatment seems to be the most effective intervention) can sometimes be the best decision.

If the literature is correct in suggesting that we cannot predict which individuals will complete suicide, then the focus of the emergency assessment of those with suicidal ideation or attempts in the PES should be to identify the factors that place people at high risk and, particularly, those factors, including illness, that may respond to treatment. Factors that place the individual at high risk may or may not be modifiable, but the assessment of risk factors helps to inform treatment planning. In general, high-risk individuals will be referred to more intensive and more secure environments. However, if hospitalization seems to be associated with a very high likelihood of disrupting outpatient treatment, emergency clinicians will have to balance treatment and security. For patients with acute risk factors who may need time to get past a crisis, safety may predominate. For patients with chronic risk factors, long-term treatment concerns may take precedence, with the recognition that a certain degree of safety will always be necessary for treatment to succeed.

Risk Factors: Fixed Versus Modifiable

In the assessment of an individual at risk for suicide, it is important to distinguish between the factors that help to identify very-high-risk individuals but that are not modifiable and the risk factors not only that place an individual at high risk but that may be modified by effective treatment. We begin this section by looking at risk factors that are relatively difficult to modify. These risk factors operate as constraints on the assessment and treatment plan.

Fixed Risk Factors

"Fixed" risk factors—those that cannot be expected to change as a consequence of successful treatment of a psychiatric disorder—include previous suicide attempts, suicidal intent at the time of the most recent attempt, sex, ethnicity, age, marital status, economic situation, and sexual orientation.

Several psychiatric measures have been created to aid in the assessment of ideation and intent. Beck et al. (1979), one of the pioneers in this field, developed a scale for suicidal ideation that looks at the intensity and pervasiveness of suicidal ideas. Mieczkowski et al. (1993) also described a scale to measure suicidal intent.

The goal of these and similar scales is to distinguish people who have a suicidal preoccupation and who make well-planned suicide attempts with intent to die from the larger group of individuals who make suicide attempts motivated more by a wish to express frustration and need than by a wish to die. This latter group is described as having made suicidal "gestures," by some authors, as opposed to suicide attempts.

Suicidal Ideation

Suicidal ideation can be thought of as both a modifiable and a fixed risk factor. Beck et al. (1999) found that the intensity of suicidal ideation at the worst point in the patient's life was a stronger predictor of suicide than hopelessness or current suicidal ideation. The extent of suicidal thoughts may be linked to a relatively persistent lowering of the psychological barriers to completed suicide or to a heritable trait. In contrast, thoughts of suicide at a given moment may not be as useful for predicting suicide, although they may be more susceptible to change with treatment.

Age, Sex, and Ethnicity

It is often said that older individuals and males are at greater risk for suicide than those who are younger and female (CDC 2000). When the data on race and ethnicity are considered (CDC 2000), older women do not generally appear to be at higher risk than younger women. The increase in risk among older individuals is largely restricted to white males and Asian males. Black males, and to a lesser extent Hispanic males, have more nearly equal risk across the age spectrum, with moderate increased risk in the early 30s and then a similar magnitude of increased risk in old age.

In the context of the data showing that, among nonwhite males, only Asian males have an increased risk when older, it is interesting to note that the increase in risk among those who are older and female is uniquely found among Asian women. By contrast, white, Hispanic, and black women tend to have lower rates of suicide in older age.

Roughly 4 times as many men as women commit suicide, although women attempt suicide twice as often as men. Historically, this difference has been ascribed to the fact that women more often make suicide attempts with poisons (such as pills) rather than with firearms. However, the percentage of women attempting suicide with firearms has significantly increased over time.

Breaking down suicide completions by sex and use or nonuse of firearms demonstrates that the increased risk of suicide among older white and Asian men correlates with a huge shift from nonfirearm suicide methods in early adulthood to firearm suicide methods in later life.

Yeates (1998), in a study of 141 suicide victims across the age spectrum by means of techniques of "psychological autopsy," found that older age was significantly associated with more determined and well-planned suicides as well as with fewer warnings of suicidal intent. Thus, the experience of many PES professionals of seeing relatively few older suicide attempters reflects the fact that older individuals are less likely to have had any contact with a mental health professional and are more likely to complete a single and lethal suicide.

An appalling sense of loss associated with the suicide of a young person, as well as data showing a significant increase in suicides among those aged 15 to 25 in the last 20 years (particularly between 1970 and 1980), has led to an increased focus on suicide among younger individuals (CDC 2000). Suicide is the sixth leading cause of death among those aged 5 to 14 and the third leading cause of death among those aged 15 to 24 (CDC 2000). The suicide rate for white males aged 15 to 24 tripled between 1950 and 1998, while the rate for white females more than doubled during that time (CDC 2000).

A study by Hawton et al. (1993) followed young people who had made suicide attempts to identify those who subsequently completed suicide. This study found that the young people who committed suicide were more likely to come from lower social classes, to have been sick enough to have previously received inpatient psychiatric treatment, to have had significant substance abuse, to have been diagnosed with personality disorders, and to have made previous suicide attempts. Nasser and Overholser (1999) also found that young people who commit suicide are, by many measures, very psychiatrically disturbed. They often have had chronic psychiatric disturbances with significant comorbidity (e.g., depression, personality disorders, substance abuse) and psychiatric disorders that extend back to early childhood. A longitudinal study following children from age 8 to age 16 found that many of the adolescents with suicidal thoughts and suicide attempts had had significant behavioral and emotional problems as early as age 8 (Sourander et al. 2001). Appleby et al. (1999a) identified a pattern of mental illness, substance abuse, social isolation, and unemployment among young people who commit suicide. Separation and rejection appear to be risk factors associated often with suicide in adolescents and young adults (Brent et al. 1993; Rich et al. 1986).

Sexual Orientation

A particularly strong risk factor for suicidal thoughts and behavior among adolescents is homosexual sexual orientation (Russell and Joyner 2001) (see below).

Herrell et al. (1999) and Fergusson et al. (1999) both found that having a gay, lesbian, or bisexual sexual orientation is associated significantly with suicidal behavior in adults as well. Fergusson et al. (1999) noted that at least 10 peer-reviewed studies found high rates of attempted suicide among young bisexual and homosexual research volunteers.

Marriage

Suicide rates are highest for those who are divorced or widowed. In 1992, the rate for divorced or widowed elderly men was 2.7 times that for married men and 1.4 times that for never-married men. The rate for divorced or widowed elderly women was 1.8 times that for married women and 1.4 times that for never-married women (CDC 2000). Later, in our discussion of modifiable risk factors, we highlight evidence that social isolation per se may be a key factor that underlies the effect of marriage.

Socioeconomic Status

The data on the relationship between suicide and socioeconomic status are mixed. The classic view was that suicide is associated with a higher socioeconomic status, but more recent population-based studies suggest a higher rate in those with a lower economic status (Taylor et al. 1998). Trouble repaying debts and an unstable financial situation often accompany suicidal ideation (Hintikka et al. 1998). An even more significant factor than economic status is the loss of employment (Kposowa 2001). For men this relationship lasts for only a few years, whereas for women the rate of suicide remains higher among the unemployed, regardless of the number of follow-up years.

History of Violence

Among risk factors that are not modifiable, it is not just suicidally destructive behavior that places individuals at higher risk. History of violent behavior of all kinds appears to increase the risk of subsequent suicide (Conner et al. 2001). Conner et al. (2001) found that violent behavior in the last year was a significant predictor of suicide and that this relationship was particularly powerful among those who had no history of alcohol abuse.

Potentially Modifiable Risk Factors

While identifying nonmodifiable risk factors helps to identify populations at risk and suggests that we intensify efforts to assess individuals who are, for instance, older white men, adolescent homosexuals, or recently unemployed men, the assessment of modifiable risk factors serves as the foundation for treatment planning in those with suicidal ideation or who have made suicide attempts.

Anxiety

A number of studies have suggested that anxiety is a major modifiable short-term risk factor for suicide. A landmark study by Fawcett (1992) of individuals who had been hospitalized for depression found that anxiety and anxiety-related symptoms, such as insomnia and difficulty in concentrating, were the most important predictors of suicide within a year of discharge. In that study, the predictors of suicide within a year were panic attacks, severe psychic anxiety, diminished concentration, global insomnia, moderate alcohol abuse, and anhedonia. The predictors of suicide after 1 year were previous attempts, hopelessness, and suicidal ideation. Busch et al. (1993) found that 13 of 14 inpatient suicides were associated with severe psychic anxiety. Our own study in the PES also identified anxiety as a major risk factor for suicide (P. L. Forster, ms. in submission).

Hopelessness and Life Satisfaction

Hopelessness was identified by Beck as a major risk factor for suicide (Beck et al. 1985). In the study by Fawcett (1992), hopelessness predicted long-term risk, but not short-term risk, of suicide. Young et al. (1996) suggested that hopelessness as a risk factor for suicide may not be as modifiable as had previously been thought. In their study, hopelessness during a depressive episode was not predictive of suicide attempts. Rather, baseline hopelessness in the absence of major depression seemed to predict future suicide attempts. Koivumaa-Honkanen et al. (2001) found that in a general population of adults, self-reported life satisfaction predicted suicide over a 20-year span; men with the highest degrees of dissatisfaction were more than 25 times as likely to commit suicide as men who were satisfied.

Access to Means

Reducing access to means of committing suicide is one of the major goals of the Surgeon General's initiative to reduce the frequency of suicide. Several lines of evidence point to the importance of assessing in an emergency evaluation the ease with which individuals can access lethal means of committing suicide. According to Brent et al. (1991), guns are two times more likely to be found in the homes of suicide completers compared with suicide attempters. More recently, Brent (2001) reviewed all the studies that have examined this relationship and concluded there is a strong relationship between firearms in the home and risk of suicide. Although those who own guns often have purchased those guns to protect themselves, only 2% of gun-related deaths in the home are the result of a home owner's shooting an intruder, whereas 83% are the result of suicide (CDC 2000). A large study that looked at the relationship between handgun purchase and death found that in the first year after the purchase of the handgun, suicide was the leading cause of death (Wintemute et al. 1999). This increase in risk appeared to be greater for women than for men.

Individuals who commit suicide by jumping off buildings or bridges are not significantly different from those who use other methods of suicide (Gunnell and Nowers 1997). The completion rate among those who jump off tall buildings is much higher than the rate among those who attempt by different means. This information, as well as the information summarized above with regard to handguns, suggests that reducing access to lethal means such as bridges without barriers and evaluating and eliminating access to guns in those who are at risk may help to prevent suicide.

Continuity of Care

One aspect of the treatment received by many individuals in the mental health system, particularly the acute mental health system, is frequent disruptions in the continuity of care. These disruptions are also a significant modifiable risk factor for suicide.

There is a significant cluster of suicides soon after discharge from psychiatric care (Goldacre et al. 1993), and two recent reviews of large numbers of suicide deaths (Appleby et al. 1999c; Burgess et al. 2000) found that disruptions in care were major preventable causes of suicide among those who had contact with the mental health system prior to their deaths. A study by Motto and Bostrom (2001) found that creating a sense of continuity of care or contact and caring for those who were resistant to seeking treatment was possible with a relatively modest effort. In his study, patients who refused to continue in treatment after evaluation but who received a letter at least four to five times a year had a significantly lower risk of suicide than similar patients who did not receive follow-up letters.

Psychiatric Illness

It is generally accepted that 90% or more of individuals who commit suicide have a serious psychiatric disorder. This finding is based on primarily retrospective, case-controlled studies of suicide. However, it is strengthened by high levels of consistency across different studies (Conwell et al. 1996; Harris and Barraclough 1997; Henriksson et al. 1993). As reviewed by Maris et al. (2000), estimates of the presence of serious psychiatric disorder across 16 studies and four decades range from 81% to 100%. The best estimate of the lifetime risk of suicide among those with depression and alcoholism (Inskip et al. 1998) puts the risk at 6%–7%, with the risk of suicide among those with schizophrenia not much lower (4%).

Data on the risk of suicide among those with bipolar disorder or personality disorders are more variable. Early studies suggested that the risk among individuals with bipolar disorder was as high as 19% (Goodwin and Jamison 1990). These studies were biased by looking over a relatively short period of time at outcomes from populations at very high risk (often looking at inpatients who were subsequently discharged from the inpatient setting). More recent studies suggest that the risk of suicide in those with bipolar disorder is either equal to (Jamison 2000) or lower than (Isometsa et al. 1994a) the risk among those with unipolar depression.

Isometsa et al. (1994b) conducted a study of all individuals who committed suicide in Finland in 1 year. The most striking findings in this study were that most of the suicide victims had major depression and that most had received no treatment for depression. Only 3% had received antidepressants at therapeutic doses, and only 7% had received weekly psychotherapy. Moreover, none of the 24 psychotic subjects had been given adequate treatment. Isometsa et al. concluded that depression not only is a major risk factor for suicide but is usually untreated, or inadequately treated, in those who commit suicide.

In Isometsa et al.'s (1994a) study of bipolar individuals who committed suicide, the majority of suicides occurred during an episode of depression (79%). In the remaining cases, as many occurred in those in a mixed state (11%) as in those who had recently recovered from a psychotic episode of mania (11%). In this group of bipolar patients, the percentage in treatment was significantly higher than in Isometsa et al.'s (1994b) study of suicides among depressed individuals. For instance, 32% had been prescribed lithium. Still, a majority of the bipolar patients had not received adequate treatment.

Among patients with mood disorders, psychotic features do not appear to significantly increase the risk of suicide (Angst and Preisig 1995; Dilsaver et al. 1994). Although the lifetime risk of suicide among individuals with schizophrenia is lower than among individuals with major depression, patients with schizophrenia appear to make more serious suicide attempts (Radomsky et al. 1999). Schizophrenic patients with predominantly negative symptoms, such as lack of will, blunted affect, or social withdrawal, have a much lower risk of suicide than those with marked suspiciousness and/or delusions (Fenton et al. 1997). Heila et al. (1997) summarized seven studies that investigated completed suicide in individuals with schizophrenia. In general, the group at highest risk appears to be young adult men in whom the illness was diagnosed within the past 10 years. Other major risk factors for suicide in schizophrenia are the presence of depressive symptoms, alcoholism, and previous suicide attempts. In Heila et al.'s (1997) study of 92 patients who completed suicide, only 1 in 10 had current suicide-commanding hallucinations, but two-thirds of the suicide completers met criteria for a depressive syndrome. Junginger (1995) found that most patients with command hallucinations ignore dangerous commands unless they are associated with delusions. Both Heila et al. (1997) and Rossau and Mortensen (1997) found that among schizophrenic patients, suicide appeared to occur most commonly following discharge from the hospital.

As reviewed by Maris et al. (2000), the rate of suicide among patients with borderline personality disorder is estimated to be between 3% and 9%—a risk comparable to that among patients with schizophrenia. The risk is greatest among those with substance abuse and depression (see below regarding the risks of suicide in complex cases).

Kramer et al. (1994) found a high correlation between suicidal ideation/suicide attempts and the diagnosis of posttraumatic stress disorder (PTSD). Moreover, Lehman et al. (1995) found a higher prevalence of completed suicides among those diagnosed with PTSD than in the general population. However, there are fewer large studies of suicide in PTSD than in major depression.

The data summarized in this subsection tend to oversimplify the diagnostic risk factors for suicide. Individuals with depression or psychotic disorders who commit suicide tend to have high rates of comorbidity with other disorders (Henriksson et al. 1993), especially substance abuse and personality disorders (Elliott et al. 1996). In one psychological autopsy study, only 12% of those who committed suicide met criteria for a single Axis I disorder; 44% had multiple Axis I disorders, 46% had contributory Axis III disorders, and between 31% and 51% met criteria for an Axis II disorder. Similarly, studies by Allebeck et al. (1991) and Duffy and Kreitman (1993) found that the combination of a personality disorder, a mood disorder, and substance use was particularly common among those who committed suicide.

The risk factors for suicide among those with substance use include the use of multiple substances, chronic substance abuse, major depression, serious medical illness, social isolation, and unemployment (Murphy et al. 1992). Motto (1980), in his prospective study of alcoholic patients, identified the presence of prior suicide attempt, the seriousness of the attempt, a negative attitude toward the interviewer, high intelligence, and having financial resources as risk factors for suicide. The risk of suicide among alcoholic individuals appears to be comparable to the risk among those with major depression (Inskip et al. 1998), and the risk of both suicide and homicide increases proportionately with alcohol intake (Klatsky and Armstrong 1993). Whereas studies of psychiatric illness and suicide find that individuals with mood disorders are more likely to commit suicide early in the course of their illness, those with alcoholism seem to be more likely to commit suicide late (Maris et al. 2000).

In summary, best estimates suggest that more than 90% of all suicides occur in those with a psychiatric illness. The most significant risk appears to be in patients with recurrent major depression or alcoholism or in patients with schizophrenia accompanied by positive symptoms (especially paranoia). Those patients who combine a mood disorder, substance abuse disorder, and personality disorder are at particularly high risk.

Social Isolation

Social isolation is a significant risk factor for suicide. Maris (1981) found that those who died from suicide were far more socially isolated across a host of domains than those who died from natural causes. Nisbet (1996) suggested that the reason that black females have the lowest rate of suicides of all race and sex groups is because they tend to have large social networks that they use when they are distressed.

Medical Illness

Medical illness appears to be an important risk factor for suicide (CDC 2000), although the relationship between having a terminal illness and planning suicide may be overestimated (Allebeck et al. 1991). Less than 1% of cancer patients die by suicide, and only 30% of cancer patients who commit suicide are considered to have a terminal condition.

By contrast, the data for AIDS patients suggest that many take medications in an effort to hasten death. In a study by Cooke et al. (1998), 12% of patients who died with AIDS had received immediately before their death an increase in medication that was intended to hasten death. Just being HIV positive is associated with, at most, a very small increase in risk of suicide (Marzuk et al. 1997). In the AIDS population, suicide appears to occur near the end of life. It should be noted that these data may be changing because of the development of antiretroviral therapy.

Other specific illnesses associated with suicide include epilepsy (Nilsson et al. 1997), cancer (Maris et al. 2000), and renal illness with dialysis.

Protective Factors

Just as there are modifiable factors that predict suicide, there are modifiable factors that protect against suicide. Factors that protect against suicide include feelings of responsibility toward family, fear of social disapproval, moral or religious objection to suicide, greater survival and coping skills, and a greater fear of suicide (Malone et al. 2000).

Risk Assessment in an Emergency Setting

Excess Mortality in Emergency Care Patients

A number of studies have examined the outcomes and long-term follow-up of individuals evaluated in an emergency setting. In a 5-year follow-up study of individuals who had been treated in hospitals following suicide attempts, Ostamo and Lonnqvist (2001) found an increased mortality in this group, not just from suicide but also from homicide and "undetermined causes." The net effect of this increased mortality was that 15% of these suicide attempters died during the 5-year follow-up period. Suicide accounted for about 40% of the excess deaths. The standard mortality ratio was highest during the first year. The authors concluded that the risk of premature death following a suicide attempt is severe.

A 14-year study of self-poisoning patients treated in the emergency unit of Helsinki University Central Hospital (Suokas and Lonnqvist 1991) also found a high mortality rate (22%). Again, about one-third of this increased mortality was due to suicide. As with the Ostamo and Lonnqvist (2001) study, risk factors for death in the Suokas and Lonnqvist study also included being male, previous suicide attempts, and a history of earlier psychiatric treatment, as well as the presence of medical illness. This study looked at psychological factors and found that the strength of the wish to die that led to the visit to the hospital was an important predictor of premature death.

A Neglected Population at Risk

In one study of emergency room patients who had deliberately harmed themselves, nearly 60% did not receive a psychiatric assessment (Hickey et al. 2001). The patients who were more likely not to have been assessed by a psychiatrist included those who had a past history of harming themselves, those who were younger (20–34 years), and those who had exhibited more difficult behavior during the time they were in the emergency room. The patients who presented between 5:00 P.M. and 9:00 A.M. were significantly less likely to be assessed than those seen between 9:00 A.M. and 5:00 P.M. Further self-harm attempts occurred in 38% of patients who had not been assessed, compared with 18% of those who had been assessed.

Risk Assessment

A suicidality assessment should be performed on every patient seen in a psychiatric emergency setting, regardless of whether the patient acknowledges suicidal ideation or has made a suicide attempt. One study found the following four questions to be a sensitive screen for significant risk of suicidality (Cooper-Patrick et al. 1994): "Has there been a period of two weeks where you have had trouble sleeping; where you have felt depressed, sad, or lost interest in things; where you have felt worthless, simple or guilty; or where you have felt hopeless for a long period of time?" Patients who acknowledge risk factors should have a further assessment for the presence of an inadequately treated psychiatric disorder that places them at risk for suicide, such as a mood disorder, psychotic disorder, substance use disorder, or personality disorder, and should be assessed for modifiable risk factors such as anxiety, insomnia, and access to means of suicide.

One approach to continuing evaluating those at risk who deny suicidal ideation is to seek to elicit negative emotion, hopelessness, and anxiety. For instance, "How bad do you feel?" might lead to the questions "Have you ever thought about death or dying?" and "What do you think the future will be like."

In a reluctant patient, it is generally more useful during a screening evaluation to look at past suicidal ideation than at ideation in the present. Individuals are more likely to acknowledge that they felt very seriously suicidal in the past than they are to express those feelings in the present, especially if they are aware that the answers may lead to unwelcome restrictions on their ability to leave the emergency setting. Moreover, as we noted, the severity of suicidal ideation at its worst point in a person's life is a better predictor of suicide than the current severity of suicidal ideation.

In evaluating an individual for suicide risk, it is also important to pay attention to one's own emotional reactions to that patient. Clinicians often report that the suicidal individual is a difficult person to take care of. Motto and Bostrom (2001) found that a negative reaction to the patient by a clinician was a significant predictor of suicide. Others have pointed to "countertransference hate" in response to the suicidal patient. Regardless of the psychodynamics, it does appear that individuals with significant suicide risk are often not identified and not aggressively treated for their illness. It is reasonable to assume that there is something very difficult for a clinician about sitting with an individual who feels so hopeless that he or she is contemplating suicide, and that there may be a subconscious wish to avoid entering the darkness of that person's experience and perhaps even a feeling that the patient's hopelessness is a reasonable response to his or her life circumstances.

Many authors have developed outlines and structured interviews for assessing suicidality. For instance, Shea (1998) proposed the CASE (Chronological Assessment of Suicide Events) approach. Thienhaus and Piasecki (1997) suggested the following elements of an assessment:

1. Establishing the patient's situation in his or her current life and living environment

2. Identifying where the patient is on the continuum of suicide risk
3. Identifying the psychiatric diagnoses
4. If the patient has suicidal thoughts, determining how realistic the patient's plan is
5. Seriously examining and evaluating potential deterrents to suicide
6. Avoiding thinking of the behavior in a derogatory way (e.g., that the patient is being "manipulative" or has made a "suicidal gesture")
7. Really imagining the place and situation that the individual will be returning to after the evaluation
8. Making a realistic assessment of the impact of your interview on the patient and your sense of connection with that person (rather than making a "no suicide" contract)
9. Getting a second opinion if you have concern
10. Not discharging an intoxicated patient

Collateral Contact

In general, there is an argument to be made for clinicians who evaluate patients at risk for suicide to make contact with collateral sources of information, such as prior providers, family, and friends (Rives 1999). Patients may not be truthful about past psychiatric illness, prior suicide attempts, or even current thoughts of suicide. Although state laws regarding confidentiality vary, a strong ethical argument can be made to breach patient confidentiality in situations in which the patient appears to be at very high risk and he or she is unwilling to authorize contact.

Interventions and Treatment

Two recent studies that looked at patients who committed suicide after prior mental health contact identified similar ways of improving treatment for this population. One study (Burgess et al. 2000) examined deaths by suicide in the state of Victoria in Australia during the period from 1989 to 1994. In this study, chart data were examined by three clinicians, who made judgments about the preventability of the suicides. The study found that among those who had prior mental health contact, a large number (49%) had contact with a mental health professional in the 4 weeks prior to death. In the retrospective assessment of the clinicians who reviewed the cases, 20% of the suicides were preventable. The key factors associated with preventability were poor staff-patient relationships, resulting in incomplete assessment, and poor assessment, leading to poor treatment of depression. Another important factor was poor continuity of care. This last finding mirrored the results of the second study done in Britain (Appleby et al. 1999b).

In Appleby et al.'s (1999c) study, the results of a 2-year review of all suicides who had had contact with mental health services in the year before death were outlined. Of the total number of suicides, roughly one-quarter had had mental health contact. In the sample with the mental health contact, 24% committed suicide within 3 months of hospital discharge, suggesting that the posthospitalization period was a time of particularly high risk. Suicide rates after hospitalization dropped rapidly during the first 5 weeks after discharge, so that the first month after discharge was the period of highest risk. Of those suicide completers who had had mental health contact, half had received services in the week before death. Just as in the previous study, the mental health teams, when asked, said that they believed about 22% of the suicides could have been prevented. Interestingly, they also specified that in 61% of the cases, at least one measure that would have significantly reduced risk. The most frequently cited interventions that might have reduced risk were interventions to improve patient compliance (29%) and those to provide closer supervision of the patients (26%).

Several of the findings cited in the study seem difficult to explain and suggest that the percentage of suicides that were judged preventable may not be a reliable estimate. The mental health teams felt that at final contact the immediate risk of suicide was absent in 30%, low in 54%, moderate in 13%, and high in only 2% of the cases. However, 16% of all the suicides occurred on inpatient units, and 5% of all the suicides occurred while the patients were on close observation for suicidality. Finally, 43% of the suicides were in the highest priority category for community care, which suggests that these patients were judged to be in need of intensive treatment for some reason.

We are skeptical about the findings of these two reviews in terms of the percentage of suicides that were "preventable" (e.g., clinicians judging that patients on constant observations were not at high risk) because of the seemingly inconsistent results and the obvious potential biases in relying on the writings or the judgments of the clinicians who were providing care.

Unfortunately, at least in the United States, legitimate concerns of clinicians about potential malpractice liability limit sharing information about how suicides with mental health contact might be prevented. In the first author's experience, after intensive review of hundreds of cases of suicide in quality improvement and forensic settings, about half of the cases seemed to have been "unexpected." In the other half, the clinicians faced an assortment of obstacles to providing effective treatment: most commonly, a lack of service integration (care being provided in multiple sites, with multiple providers, without good continuity); often, a failure to adequately treat all the identified problems (e.g., substance abuse problems comorbid with other disorders, anxiety, or insomnia symptoms); and in some cases, concerns about how to involve family members or other significant others in working with a patient at risk in the evaluation or treatment of a patient. Some of these obstacles could not have been overcome by the individual clinician (legal, or "systems," issues), but that does not mean that those suicides were not potentially preventable.

Another study by Appleby et al. (1999b) examined all of the patients who committed suicide in Greater Manchester following a psychiatric hospitalization and matched this group of patients with patients who were discharged from the inpatient unit but who did not commit suicide. Those who committed suicide were four times more likely to have had their care reduced at the final appointment before their death. In this study, only one-third of the patients who committed suicide had an identifiable case manager at the time of death. This finding was no different from what was found for the group of patients who did not commit suicide, suggesting that there might have been a failure to provide intensive treatment to this group of patients. It is interesting to wonder about the transference and countertransference implications of a reduction in care immediately preceding suicide.

The importance of the clinical relationship as a mediating factor in suicide is illustrated by a study by Granboulan et al. (2001). In this study, 167 adolescents who had been hospitalized following a suicide attempt were examined to determine what factors were associated with higher compliance with follow-up care. Two important factors were the amount of time that the adolescent met with the psychiatrist while hospitalized and the duration of hospitalization. Just as clearly, the subjective factors that are the hardest to evaluate retrospectively (e.g., therapeutic alliance, empathy) are significant in the outcome for patients at risk.

Immediate Treatment Interventions

Treatment interventions can be somewhat artificially divided into those that have some possibility of changing the patient's suicidal ideation within the first few days after evaluation and those that take longer to be effective. Of particular interest to the psychiatric emergency clinician are those interventions that may have some immediate benefit.

Anxiety

Severe anxiety, agitation, and panic attacks are correlated with acute suicide risk, and denial of suicidal ideation in a patient who is extremely anxious should not be taken at face value (Fawcett et al. 1990; Hall et al. 1999; Schnyder et al. 1999). Patients with significant anxiety who are at risk for suicide should have that anxiety aggressively treated. Similarly, those with other, possibly related symptoms, such as insomnia, should have aggressive treatment for those conditions. Extreme anxiety or paranoia should always be treated in those at risk and may be grounds for intensive treatment by itself. Clinicians are often uncomfortable with prescribing medications for anxiolysis and insomnia because of concern about abuse of the medications. Given the high rate of suicide in these patients, it is clear that the risk of abuse needs to be balanced with the importance of providing effective treatment for anxiety.

Other Issues

Clinicians should pay attention to the following issues in making immediate treatment plans:

1. *First, do no harm.* Do not provide the patient with medications that are potentially toxic in overdose.
2. *Remove access to means of committing suicide.* It is extremely important to assess whether a patient who is suicidal has access to a weapon. Studies find that about half of all Americans have ready access to a gun, and easy access to a gun clearly is associated with an increased risk of suicide. Family members can be asked to take charge of a weapon in the house, if necessary.
3. *Offer the patient hope.* We have already cited several studies to suggest that continuity of care and the quality and intensity of the treatment relationship are important factors that reduce suicide. In the emergency setting, the clinician should try to help patients see that their problems can be solved and that the clinician is personally willing and able to help. In this context, countertransference reactions need to be monitored, since a clinician who is feeling more empathy for a patient is more likely to be able to convey that message.

An intriguing study by Gustafson et al. (1993) found a significant relationship between follow-up to treatment and objective measurements of quality of care and of patient satisfaction. The key process variables that predicted follow-up were 1) being adequately involved with the patient, 2) obtaining a complete patient history, 3) performing appropriate laboratory tests, 4) developing an adequate diagnostic formulation, and 5) taking appropriate action. Included in adequate involvement with the patient were the identification of the patient's social support and contact with that social support and the establishment of contact with a therapist. In a busy PES, it may be difficult to do all these things, but this study suggests that the more careful the assessment, the more likely patients will be to comply with treatment.

Hospitalization

One of the important questions facing a clinician who is planning treatment for a suicidal patient is the question of whether to hospitalize. Several studies suggest that clinicians may be overly reliant on hospitalization as an intervention. For instance, Schnyder and Valach (1997) found that many of the patients who had attempted suicide were better integrated occupationally and socially in their communities than other patients evaluated in an emergency setting. Relatives and friends were more frequently involved in the consultation. Despite this, these patients were more frequently hospitalized. The authors suggest that junior physicians should be encouraged not to reflexively hospitalize patients who attempt suicide.

In a study by Waterhouse and Platt (1990), patients who had made suicide attempts were randomly assigned to a group that was admitted (38 cases) and a group that was discharged home (39 cases). In this relatively small study, there was no significant difference in outcome between the groups, both of which showed overall improvement. Rosenbluth et al. (1995) discussed some of the ethical issues involved in treatment planning with the suicidal patient. They pointed out that, in some cases, respecting a patient's autonomy may allow a better clinical relationship to develop and that, consequently, hospitalization may be a less effective intervention.

Zealberg and Santos (1996) suggested that referral of a suicidal patient to inpatient care should always occur if the method of attempt involved high lethality (e.g., firearms, hanging, jumping); if the patient has specific plans, means, and intent to commit suicide; if the patient continues to express a wish to die after the attempt; or if there is no social support network available. We certainly agree with the need to be very cautious in the assessment of patients with these characteristics, but we still feel that it is appropriate to temper rules like this with clinical judgment about what form of treatment is the most likely to be effective. In systems where a clinical relationship established in the emergency setting can continue afterward, and particularly where there is good availability for phone contact should symptoms worsen, more "risks" can, and probably should, be taken in terms of outpatient referral. Further, there are some people who learned that suicidal behavior, such as ideation and "gestures," will lead to inpatient hospitalization and who seek hospitalization for nontreatment purposes. With these individuals, if they are well known to the clinician, and if their behavior is unchanged (not worsened in severity), outpatient referral may be appropriate. These persons are often allowed to "wait" in the PES until they are no longer suicidal.

Psychosocial Treatment

There is mixed information regarding the potential of psychotherapeutic intervention to reduce the risk of suicide. In a study by Guthrie et al. (2001), 119 individuals who had taken an overdose were randomized to usual care or to four sessions of brief psychodynamic interpersonal therapy delivered in the patient's home. This very short-term intervention was associated with a significant reduction in suicidal ideation at 6 months (an 8-point reduction in the treatment group versus a 1.5-point reduction in the control group). Those who participated were more satisfied with the treatment and less likely to report further attempts at self-harm.

In contrast, a study by Van Der Sande et al. (1997b) found that an intensive inpatient and community intervention program for suicidal attempters was no more effective than "care as usual." In a separate article, Van Der Sande et al. (1997a) completed a meta-analysis of all of the studies looking at psychosocial interventions in those at risk of suicide. In this large analysis, they found that "crisis intervention," as well as guaranteed inpatient treatment, did not result in any significant reduction in suicide attempts. On the other hand, the combined results of four studies looking at cognitive-behavioral therapies found a significant effect in reducing suicide attempts. From this study and the Guthrie study, it appears that psychologically sophisticated and manualized treatments may be quite effective in the immediate reduction of suicide intentionality but that just providing "crisis intervention" may not.

Psychosis

Finally, in considering interventions for immediate treatment, it is worth noting the importance of providing effective treatment for psychotic individuals with depressive symptoms. However, there is clear evidence that many of the atypical antipsychotics are more effective than typical antipsychotics in reducing depressive and anxiety symptoms in patients who are psychotic (see section on long-term treatment later in this chapter), and so those medications should be used in preference to typical antipsychotics. In addition, electroconvulsive therapy (ECT), although not readily available in many communities, can be effective in treating severe depression almost immediately and can even be done on an outpatient basis.

Long-Term Treatment Considerations

A study by Gustafson et al. (1993), in which the quality of the treatment plan and of the diagnostic evaluation was correlated with treatment compliance, emphasizes the importance, even in an emergency setting, of identifying psychiatric disorders that contribute to suicide risk. Obviously, the patient is going to be much more hopeful when given a clear diagnosis and a thoughtful explanation of how appropriate medications can be expected to reduce their suffering than in the context of a referral for unspecified treatment from an unknown provider.

Antidepressants

Effective treatment of major depression is often not provided to patients who commit suicide. Since depressive disorders are associated with half of all suicides, this failure is remarkable. Perhaps one context for this is the fact that tricyclic antidepressants (TCAs) were often associated with overdoses. Studies by Freemantle et al. (1994) and Crome (1993) identified major differences in toxicity between the older TCAs and the selective serotonin reuptake inhibitors (SSRIs). Amoxapine and desipramine had particularly high risk of toxicity and death in these studies, but all the older TCAs were dangerous. By contrast, maprotiline and trazodone had relatively low risks, and the SSRIs had essentially no risk.

Another controversy that may have discouraged people from prescribing antidepressants in an emergency setting is the suggestion that there is a short-term increase in suicide risk immediately after beginning antidepressants. Although there are many case reports of such increased risk, several studies found that antidepressants reduce suicidal ideation even early in treatment (Montgomery et al. 1995; Tollefson et al. 1994). Leon et al. (1999), in a study of 643 patients treated with fluoxetine, found a reduction in suicide attempts in the treated patients, despite the presence of severe psychopathology before treatment. Still, Muller-Oerlinghausen and Berghofer (1999) cited the weaknesses in the literature and recommended caution in prescribing medications that may induce akathisia, such as SSRIs. Perhaps a way out of this apparent bind is to use a combination of an SSRI and clonazepam. Smith et al. (1998) found a significantly faster response to the antidepressant, as well as a more powerful long-term effect, associated with this combination. If we treat anxiety and insomnia, and incidentally provide prophylaxis against akathisia or activation side effects by adding an anxiolytic to an antidepressant, we may be more effective in treating depressed patients in an emergency setting.

Isacsson et al. (1997) found that the increased use of antidepressants in Sweden between 1990 and 1994 was associated with a significant decrease in suicide rates. Whether this was a cause or an effect is unknown, but they suggested that the acute toxicity of antidepressants is of minor importance compared with the need to provide more aggressive treatment for depressed suicidal patients.

Mood Stabilizers

Several studies of patients with bipolar disorder who committed suicide found a relatively low rate of treatment with therapeutic levels of mood stabilizers. Isometsa et al. (1994a) found that only 16% of bipolar patients who committed suicide were receiving therapeutic doses of lithium. Although there is mixed evidence for the ability of other mood stabilizers to reduce suicide risk, there is compelling evidence that lithium treatment does reduce the risk. Tondo et al. (1998) found that lithium maintenance was associated with a marked reduction of life-threatening suicide attempts. Tondo et al. (1997) identified 28 studies with 17,294 patients with bipolar disorder. In their analysis of these studies, these authors concluded that there was a consistent reduction of suicide in patients treated with lithium.

Atypical Antipsychotics

Several studies have also found significant reductions in suicide rates among patients treated with clozapine. Meltzer and Okayli (1995) found that patients with neuroleptic-resistant schizophrenia who were treated with clozapine showed a marked reduction (86%) in suicide attempts and suicides. Meltzer (1998) cited studies that compared suicide deaths in patients in the clozapine registry with patients before clozapine was initiated and while taking clozapine. These studies found that the incidence of suicide during clozapine treatment was one-fifth the incidence of suicide prior to clozapine treatment.

Although the data are less compelling, there is evidence that olanzapine reduces depression and anxiety symptoms more than haloperidol (Tollefson et al. 1998). Marder et al. (1997) cited evidence for greater improvements on anxiety and depression scales in schizophrenic patients treated with risperidone compared with patients treated with haloperidol. By contrast, Palmer et al. (1999) reviewed several uncontrolled studies that suggested an increased risk of suicide after treatment with typical antipsychotics was initiated. Findings from these studies, however, may have been confounded by the fact that patients were often released from the hospital at roughly the same time that they began taking typical antipsychotics. Palmer et al. (1999) also examined studies which suggested that among those treated with typical agents, there was no effect on suicidality or perhaps a slight reduction in risk. In these studies, very low and very high doses of typical antipsychotics did appear to be associated with an increased risk. Thus, it is reasonable to suggest that increased use of atypical antipsychotics may lead to further reductions in suicide.

Treatment Planning

The information that we have cited in the foregoing subsections is generally consistent with the position that we have taken that ensuring effective treatment of psychiatric disorders is the key issue that should be the focus of treatment planning in the emergency service. At the very least, the studies on lithium and clozapine suggest that potentially toxic medications may not be contraindicated in treating severely ill and suicidal patients.

Medical-Legal Issues

Just as suicide has markedly shaped the practice of emergency psychiatry, the threat of malpractice has had a profound impact on how we treat suicidal patients. The standard for malpractice is that the clinician must exercise the degree of knowledge and skill in diagnosis and treatment ordinarily possessed by his or her peers. Failures commonly associated with malpractice actions (Bongar et al. 1998) include the following:

- Failure to adequately evaluate or treat the patient pharmacologically
- Failure to specify under what criteria the patient might be hospitalized
- Failure to establish proper boundaries in therapy
- Failure to obtain consultation
- Failure to evaluate risk adequately
- Failure to obtain prior records, diagnose, or conduct a mental status examination
- Failure to establish a treatment plan

Although the results of individual malpractice cases can be very confusing, it appears that the largest risk of malpractice is associated with inadequate documentation. There is not really credible scientific evidence to suggest that clinicians, in individual cases, are effective at judging the risk of suicide. Also, juries are often reluctant to absolve patients from some responsibility for their actions. Thus, clinicians who adequately assess and document their assessment and who provide a coherent rationale for their treatment plan, even when their treatment plan involves a less restrictive alternative such as intensive outpatient care, are unlikely to be found to have committed malpractice. This is particularly true in cases in which the clinician obtained consultation contemporaneously.

The fear of malpractice action may needlessly constrain the PES clinician from carefully thinking through the most effective way to provide treatment for the patient's underlying disorder. This concern may actually have a stultifying effect on the clinician, reducing the assessment in an emergency setting to a review of risk factors and a decision whether or not to admit the patient, rather than encouraging a process of careful assessment and engagement of the patient and conveying a sense of hope that comes from a thoughtful treatment plan and a clear diagnosis.

Conclusion

Suicide is almost always the catastrophic result of inadequately treated psychiatric illness. Sometimes this outcome is inherent in the nature of the mental health treatment system or of the laws that society has established to balance the value of individual autonomy and the provision of effective treatment. Sometimes the outcome is the result of inadequate assessment, an inadequate treatment plan, or inadequate treatment. Still, working with patients at risk of suicide is something that is poorly rewarded in most systems of care, and malpractice law is generally a destructive way of perfecting the system that cares for the sickest patients.

Clinicians working in an emergency setting should make vigorous efforts to assess those individuals at risk, to identify inadequately treated psychiatric disorders, to ensure continuity of care, and to treat those symptoms and conditions that may be quickly reversible, such as anxiety, insomnia, and self-imposed social isolation. They must also be watchful of their own emotional reactions to the individual patient, or to the stress of the work environment, and seek to convey hope to those without hope.

Systems of care need to develop better linkages between acute care and aftercare. They also need to ensure adequate treatment for complex cases in which patients have multiple diagnoses (including mood disorders and substance abuse).

Researchers should be encouraged to explore not just the easily verifiable correlates of suicide but also the harder-to-identify but equally important subjective factors, including those related to relationships with caregivers.

References

Allebeck P, Allgulander C, Henningsohn L, et al: Causes of death in a cohort of 50,465 young men: validity of recorded suicide as underlying cause of death. Scand J Soc Med 19(4):242–247, 1991

Allgulander C, Fisher LD: Clinical predictors of completed suicide and repeated self-poisoning in 8895 self-poisoning patients. Eur Arch Psychiatry Neurol Sci 239(4):270–276, 1990

Angst J, Preisig M: Outcome of a clinical cohort of unipolar, bipolar and schizoaffective patients: results of a prospective study from 1959 to 1985. Schweiz Arch Neurol Psychiatr 146(1):17–23, 1995

Appleby L, Cooper J, Amos T, et al: Psychological autopsy study of suicides by people aged under 35. Br J Psychiatry 75:168–74, 1999a

Appleby L, Dennehy JA, Thomas CS, et al: Aftercare and clinical characteristics of people with mental illness who commit suicide: a case-control study. Lancet 353(9162):1397–1400, 1999b

Appleby L, Shaw J, Amos T, et al: Suicide within 12 months of contact with mental health services: national clinical survey. Br Med J 318 (7193):1235–1239, 1999c

Baca-Garcia E, Diaz-Sastre C, Basurte E, et al: A prospective study of the paradoxical relationship between impulsivity and lethality of suicide attempts. J Clin Psychiatry 62(7):560–564, 2001

Beck AT, Kovacs M, Weissman A: Assessment of suicidal intention: the Scale for Suicide Ideation. J Consult Clin Psychol 47(2):343–352, 1979

Beck AT, Steer RA, Kovacs M, et al: Hopelessness and eventual suicide: a 10-year prospective study of patients hospitalized with suicidal ideation. Am J Psychiatry 142(5):559–563, 1985

Beck AT, Brown GK, Steer RA: Suicide ideation at its worst point: a predictor of eventual suicide in psychiatric outpatients. Suicide Life Threat Behav 29(1):1–9, 1999

Bongar B, Berman A, Maris R, et al: Risk Management With Suicidal Patients. New York, Guilford, 1998

Brent DA: Firearms and suicide. Ann N Y Acad Sci 932:225–239 [discussion: 239–240], 2001

Brent DA, Perper JA, Allman CJ, et al: The presence and accessibility of firearms in the homes of adolescent suicides: a case-control study. JAMA 266(21):2989–2995, 1991

Brent DA, Perper JA, Moritz G, et al: Psychiatric risk factors for adolescent suicide: a case-control study. J Am Acad Child Adolesc Psychiatry 32:521–529, 1993

Burgess P, Pirkis J, Morton J, et al: Lessons from a comprehensive clinical audit of users of psychiatric services who committed suicide. Psychiatr Serv 51(12):1555–1560, 2000

Busch KA, Clark DC, Fawcett J, et al: Clinical features of inpatient suicide. Psychiatric Annals 23:256–262, 1993

Centers for Disease Control and Prevention: Deaths: Final data for 1998. National Vital Statistic Reports 48(11), 2000

Conner KR, Cox C, Duberstein PR, et al: Violence, alcohol, and completed suicide: a case-control study. Am J Psychiatry 158(10):1701–1705, 2001

Conwell Y, Duberstein PR, Cox C, et al: Relationships of age and Axis I diagnosis in victims of completed suicide: a psychological autopsy study. Am J Psychiatry 153:1001–1008, 1996

Cooke M, Gourlay L, Collette L, et al: Informal caregivers and the intention to hasten AIDS-related death. Arch Intern Med 158(1):69–75, 1998

Cooper-Patrick L, Crum RM, Ford DE: Identifying suicidal ideation in general medical patients. JAMA 272(22):1757–1762, 1994

Crome P: The toxicity of drugs used for suicide. Acta Psychiatr Scand Suppl 371:33–37, 1993

Dhossche DM: Suicidal behavior in psychiatric emergency room patients. South Med J 93(3):310–314, 2000

Dilsaver SC, Chen YW, Swann AC, et al: Suicidality in patients with pure and depressive mania. Am J Psychiatry 151(9):1312–1315, 1994

Duffy J, Kreitman N: Risk factors for suicide and undetermined death among in-patient alcoholics in Scotland. Addiction 88(6):757–766, 1993

Earle KA, Forquer SL, Volo AM, et al: Characteristics of outpatient suicides. Hosp Community Psychiatry 45(2):123–126, 1994

Elliott AJ, Pages KP, Russo J, et al: A profile of medically serious suicide attempts. J Clin Psychiatry 57(12):567–571, 1996

Fawcett J: Suicide risk factors in depressive disorders and in panic disorder. J Clin Psychiatry 53(3, suppl):9–13, 1992

Fawcett J, Scheftner WA, Fogg L: Time-related predictors of suicide in major affective disorder. Am J Psychiatry 147(9):1189–1194, 1990

Fenton WS, McGlashan TH, Vicort BJ, et al: Symptoms, subtype, and suicidality in patients with schizophrenia spectrum disorders. Am J Psychiatry 154(2):199–204, 1997

Fergusson DM, Horwood LJ, Beautrais AL: Is sexual orientation related to mental health problems and suicidality in young people? Arch Gen Psychiatry 56(10):876–880, 1999

Freemantle N, House A, Song F, et al: Prescribing selective serotonin reuptake inhibitors as strategy for prevention of suicide. BMJ 309 (6949):249–253, 1994

Goldacre M, Seagroatt V, Hawton K: Suicide after discharge from psychiatric inpatient care. Lancet 342(8866):283–286, 1993

Goodwin FK, Jamison KR: Manic-Depressive Illness. New York, Oxford University Press. 1990

Granboulan V, Roudot-Thoraval F, Lemerle S, et al: Predictive factors of post-discharge follow-up care among adolescent suicide attempters. Acta Psychiatr Scand 104(1):31–36, 2001

Gunnell D, Nowers M: Suicide by jumping. Acta Psychiatr Scand 96(1): 1–6, 1997

Gustafson DH, Sainfort F, Johnson SW, et al: Measuring quality of care in psychiatric emergencies: construction and evaluation of a Bayesian index. Health Serv Res 28(2):131–58, 1993

Guthrie E, Kapur N, Mackway-Jones K, et al: Randomised controlled trial of brief psychological intervention after deliberate self poisoning. BMJ 323(7305):135–138, 2001

Hall RC, Platt DE, Hall RC: Suicide risk assessment: a review of risk factors for suicide in 100 patients who made severe suicide attempts. Evaluation of suicide risk in a time of managed care. Psychosomatics 40(1):18–27, 1999

Harris EC, Barraclough B: Suicide as an outcome for mental disorders: a meta-analysis. Br J Psychiatry 170:205–228, 1997

Hawton K, Fagg J, Platt S, et al: Factors associated with suicide after parasuicide in young people. Br Med J 306(6893)1641–1644. 1993

Heila H, Isometsa ET, Henriksson MM, et al: Suicide and schizophrenia: a nationwide psychological autopsy study on age- and sex-specific clinical characteristics of 92 suicide victims with schizophrenia. Am J Psychiatry 154(9):1235–1242, 1997

Henriksson MM, Aro HM, Marttunen MJ, et al: Mental disorders and comorbidity in suicide. Am J Psychiatry 150(6):935–940, 1993

Herrell R, Goldberg J, True WR, et al: Sexual orientation and suicidality: a co-twin control study in adult men. Arch Gen Psychiatry 56(10): 867–874, 1999

Hickey L, Hawton K, Fagg J, et al: Deliberate self-harm patients who leave the accident and emergency department without a psychiatric assessment: a neglected population at risk of suicide. J Psychosom Res 50(2):87–93, 2001

Hintikka J, Kontula O, Saarinen P, et al: Debt and suicidal behaviour in the Finnish general population. Acta Psychiatr Scand 98(6):493–496, 1998

Inskip HM, Harris EC, Barraclough B: Lifetime risk of suicide for affective disorder, alcoholism and schizophrenia. Br J Psychiatry 172:35–37, 1998

Isacsson G, Holmgren P, Druid H, et al: The utilization of antidepressants—a key issue in the prevention of suicide: an analysis of 5281 suicides in Sweden during the period 1992–1994. Acta Psychiatr Scand 96(2):94–100, 1997

Isometsa ET, Henriksson MM, Aro HM, et al: Suicide in bipolar disorder in Finland. Am J Psychiatry 151(7):1020–1024, 1994a

Isometsa ET, Henriksson MM, Aro HM, et al: Suicide in major depression. Am J Psychiatry 151(4):530–536, 1994b

Isometsa ET, Heikkinen ME, Marttunen MJ, et al: The last appointment before suicide: is suicide intent communicated? Am J Psychiatry 152(6): 919–922, 1995

Jamison KR: Suicide and bipolar disorder. J Clin Psychiatry 61 (9, suppl): 47–51, 2000

Junginger J: Command hallucinations and the prediction of dangerousness. Psychiatr Serv 51(12):911–914, 1995

Kessler RC, Borges G, Walters EE: Prevalence of and risk factors for lifetime suicide attempts in the National Comorbidity Survey. Arch Gen Psychiatry 56:617–626, 1999

Klatsky AL, Armstrong MA: Alcohol use, other traits, and risk of unnatural death: a prospective study. Alcohol Clin Exp Res 17(6):1156–1162, 1993

Koivumaa-Honkanen H, Honkanen R, Viinamaki H, et al: Life satisfaction and suicide: a 20-year follow-up study. Am J Psychiatry 158(3): 433–439, 2001

Kposowa AJ: Unemployment and suicide: a cohort analysis of social factors predicting suicide in the US National Longitudinal Mortality Study. Psychol Med 31(1):127–138, 2001

Kramer T, Lindy J, Green B, et al: The comorbidity of post-traumatic stress disorder and suicidality in Vietnam veterans. Suicide Life Threat Behav 24:58–67, 1994

Lehman L, McCormick R, McCracken L: Suicidal behavior among patients in the VA health care system. Psychiatr Serv 46:1069–1071, 1995

Leon AC, Keller MB, Warshaw MG, et al: Prospective study of fluoxetine treatment and suicidal behavior in affectively ill subjects. Am J Psychiatry 156(2):195–201, 1999

Malone KM, Szanto K, Corbitt EM, et al: Clinical assessment versus research methods in the assessment of suicidal behavior. Am J Psychiatry 152(11):1601–1607, 1995

Malone KM, Oquendo MA, Haas GL, et al: Protective factors against suicidal acts in major depression: reasons for living. Am J Psychiatry 157(7):1084–1088, 2000

Marder SR, Davis JM, Chouinard G: The effects of risperidone on the five dimensions of schizophrenia derived by factor analysis: combined results of the North American trials. J Clin Psychiatry 58(12): 538–546, 1997

Maris RW: Pathway to Survive: A Survey of Self-Destructive Behaviors. Baltimore, MD, Johns Hopkins University Press, 1981

Maris RW, Berman AL, Maltsberger JT, et al: Assessment and Prediction of Suicide. New York, Guilford, 1992

Maris RW, Berman AL, Silverman MM: Comprehensive Textbook of Suicidology. London, Guilford, 2000

Marzuk PM, Tardiff K, Leon AC, et al: HIV seroprevalence among suicide victims in New York City, 1991–1993. Am J Psychiatry 154(12): 1720–1725, 1997

Meltzer HY: Suicide in schizophrenia: risk factors and clozapine treatment. J Clin Psychiatry 59 (3, suppl):15–20, 1998

Meltzer HY, Okayli G: Reduction of suicidality during clozapine treatment of neuroleptic-resistant schizophrenia: impact on risk-benefit assessment. Am J Psychiatry 152(2):183–190, 1995

Mieczkowski TA, Sweeney JA, Haas GL, et al: Factor composition of the Suicide Intent Scale. Suicide Life Threat Behav 23(1):37–45, 1993

Montgomery SA, Dunner DL, Dunbar GC: Reduction of suicidal thoughts with paroxetine in comparison with reference antidepressants and placebo. Eur Neuropsychopharmacol 5(1):5–13, 1995

Motto JA: Suicide risk factor in alcohol abuse. Suicide Life Threat Behav 10:230–238, 1980

Motto JA, Bostrom A: Empirical indicators of near-term suicide risk. Crisis 11(1):52–59, 1990a

Motto JA, Bostrom AG: Models of suicide risk. Crisis 11(2):37–47, 1990b

Motto JA, Bostrom AG: A randomized controlled trial of postcrisis suicide prevention. Psychiatr Serv 52:828–833, 2001

Muller-Oerlinghausen B, Berghofer A: Antidepressants and suicidal risk. J Clin Psychiatry 60 (2, suppl):94–99 [discussion: 111–116], 1999

Murphy GE, Wetzel RD, Robins E, et al: Multiple risk factors predict suicide in alcoholism. Arch Gen Psychiatry 49(6):459–463, 1992

Nasser EH, Overholser JC: Assessing varying degrees of lethality in depressed adolescent suicide attempters. Acta Psychiatr Scand 99(6): 123–131, 1999

Nilsson L, Tomson T, Farahmand BY, et al: Cause-specific mortality in epilepsy: a cohort study of more than 9,000 patients once hospitalized for epilepsy. Epilepsia 38(10):1059–1061, 1997

Nisbet PA: Protective factors for suicidal black females. Suicide Life Threat Behav 26(4):325–341, 1996

Obafunwa J, Busuttil A: Clinical contact preceding suicide. The Fellowship of Postgraduate Medicine 70:428–432, 1994

Ostamo A, Lonnqvist J: Excess mortality of suicide attempters. Soc Psychiatry Psychiatr Epidemiol 36(1):29–35, 2001

Palmer DD, Henter ID, Wyatt RJ: Do antipsychotic medications decrease the risk of suicide in patients with schizophrenia? J Clin Psychiatry 60 (2, suppl):100–103 [discussion: 111–116], 1999

Pokorny AD: Prediction of suicide in psychiatric patients: report of a prospective study. Arch Gen Psychiatry 40:249–257, 1983

Radomsky ED, Haas GL, Mann JJ, et al: Suicidal behavior in patients with schizophrenia and other psychotic disorders. Am J Psychiatry 156(10):1590–1595, 1999

Rich CL, Young JG, Fowler RC. San Diego Suicide Study, I: young vs old subjects. Arch Gen Psychiatry 43:524–527, 1986

Rives W: Emergency department assessment of suicidal patients. Psychiatr Clin North Am 22(4): 779–787, 1999

Rosenbluth M, Kleinman I, Lowy F: Suicide: the interaction of clinical and ethical issues. Psychiatr Serv 46(9):919–921, 1995

Rossau CD, Mortensen PB: Risk factors for suicide in patients with schizophrenia: nested case-control study. Br J Psychiatry 171:355–359, 1997

Russell ST, Joyner K: Adolescent sexual orientation and suicide risk: evidence from a national study. Am J Public Health 91(8):1276–1281, 2001

Schnyder U, Valach L: Suicide attempters in a psychiatric emergency room population. Gen Hosp Psychiatry 19(2):119–129, 1997

Schnyder U, Valach L, Bichsel K, et al: Attempted suicide: do we understand the patients' reasons? Gen Hosp Psychiatry 21(1):62–69, 1999

Shea SC: The chronological assessment of suicide events: a practical interviewing strategy for the elicitation of suicidal ideation. J Clin Psychiatry 59 (suppl 20):58–72, 1998

Smith WT, Londborg PD, Glaudin V, et al: Short-term augmentation of fluoxetine with clonazepam in the treatment of depression: a double-blind study. Am J Psychiatry 155(10):1339–1345, 1998

Sourander A, Helstela L, Haavisto A, et al: Suicidal thoughts and attempts among adolescents: a longitudinal 8-year follow-up study. J Affect Disord 63(1–3):59–66, 2001

Suokas J: Long term risk factors for suicide mortality after attempted suicide—findings of a 14-year follow up study. Acta Psychiatr Scand 104:117–121, 2001

Suokas J, Lonnqvist J: Selection of patients who attempted suicide for psychiatric consultation. Acta Psychiatr Scand 83(3):179–82, 1991

Taylor R, Morrell S, Slaytor E, et al: Suicide in urban New South Wales, Australia 1985–1994: socio-economic and migrant interactions. Soc Sci Med 47(11):1677–1686, 1998

Thienhaus OJ, Piasecki M: Assessment of suicide risk. Psychiatr Serv 48(3):293–294, 1997

Tollefson GD, Rampey AH Jr, Beasley CM Jr: Absence of a relationship between adverse events and suicidality during pharmacotherapy for depression. J Clin Psychopharmacol 14(3):163–169, 1994

Tollefson GD, Sanger TM, Lu Y, et al: Depressive signs and symptoms in schizophrenia: a prospective blinded trial of olanzapine and haloperidol. Arch Gen Psychiatry 55(3):250–258, 1998

Tondo L, Jamison KR, Baldessarini RJ: Effect of lithium maintenance on suicidal behavior in major mood disorders. Ann N Y Acad Sci 836:339–351, 1997

Tondo L, Baldessarini RJ, Hennen J, et al: Lithium treatment and risk of suicidal behavior in bipolar disorder patients. J Clin Psychiatry 59(8):405–414, 1998

U.S. Public Health Service: The Surgeon General's Call to Action to Prevent Suicide. Washington, DC, U.S. Public Health Service, 1999

Van Der Sande R, Buskens E, Allart E, et al: Psychosocial intervention following suicide attempt: a systematic review of treatment interventions. Acta Psychiatr Scand 96(1):43–50, 1997a

Van Der Sande R, van Rooijen L, Buskens E, et al: Intensive in-patient and community intervention versus routine care after attempted suicide: a randomised controlled intervention study. Br J Psychiatry 171:35–41, 1997b

Waterhouse J, Platt S: General hospital admission in the management of parasuicide: a randomised controlled trial. Br J Psychiatry 156:236–242, 1990

Welch SS: A review of the literature on the epidemiology of parasuicide in the general population. Psychiatr Serv 52:368–375, 2001

Wintemute GJ, Parham CA, Beaumont JJ: Mortality among recent purchasers of handguns. N Engl J Med 341(21):1583–1589, 1999

Yeates C: Age differences in behaviors leading to completed suicide. Am J Geriatr Psychiatry 6:122–126, 1998

Young MA, Fogg LF, Scheftner W, et al: Stable trait components of hopelessness: baseline and sensitivity to depression. J Abnorm Psychol 105(2):155–165, 1996

Zealberg JJ, Santos AB: Comprehensive Emergency Mental Health Care. New York, WW Norton, 1996

Chapter 4

Emergency Treatment of Agitation and Aggression

J. P. Lindenmayer, M.D.
Martha Crowner, M.D.
Victoria Cosgrove, B.A.

Definitions

Agitation and aggression are nonspecific constellations of behaviors that can be seen in a number of different clinical conditions. They are best seen as *transnosological syndromes,* meaning that one can find these clusters of behaviors present in a number of different psychiatric disorders. Behavioral signs of agitation include restlessness, fidgetiness, hyperactivity, and jitteriness. All these terms describe a state of poorly organized and aimless psychomotor activity that stems from physical or mental unease (Sachdev and Kruk 1996). Motor restlessness, hyperactivity, heightened responsivity to external or internal stimuli, irritability, and inappropriate verbal or motor activity that is often purposeless and repetitive are the hallmark of agitation. In addition, vegetative signs, such as disturbed sleep pattern, are often present. Patients may complain of a subjective component in terms of inner restlessness, inability to sit still, and hyperactivity. Agitation usually presents with a fluctuating course that can change rapidly over time.

Attempts have been made to classify subtypes of agitation. Cohen-Mansfield and Billig (1986) distinguished an aggressive physical component (e.g., fighting, throwing, grabbing, destroying items), an aggressive verbal component (e.g., cursing, screaming), a nonaggressive physical component (e.g., pacing), and a nonaggressive verbal component (e.g., constant questioning, chatting). All are, by and large, inappropriate on the basis of social standards.

Moyer (1976, p. 2) defined aggressive behavior as "overt behavior involving intent to inflict noxious stimulation or to behave destructively towards another organism." Two types of aggressive behaviors are often differentiated. *Impulsive* violence is usually a hair-trigger response to a stimulus that results in an agitated state and culminates in an exaggerated aggressive response. This is, therefore, the type of aggression usually seen in the mentally ill and is a frequent result of agitated states. In contrast, *premeditated* violence, often predatory in nature, is more deliberately planned and executed.

Diagnostic Considerations

In this section, we review the presentation of agitation and aggression across diagnostic groups and consider the ways in which the context, precipitants, and severity of assaults are typically affected by psychopathology (for review, see Volavka 1995; Crowner 2000; Monahan et al. 2001). It is important for clinicians to be familiar with the disorders that are particularly associated with violence. The more specific the diagnostic assessment is, the more specific the treatment can be.

Clinicians assess individuals who may be agitated and violent in various settings, including emergency rooms, inpatient wards, and outpatient clinics. Violence in the community often presents differently and may also need to be assessed differently than institutional violence. Substance abuse is more commonly associated with violence occurring in the community, where substances are freely available. Studies consistently find that substance abuse increases the risk of violent behavior and that comorbidity of substance abuse with another psychiatric disorder presents a still greater risk (Steadman et al. 1978). Weapons are more freely available in the community, so serious injuries and legal consequences are more common.

Various functions such as perception, judgment, planning, mood, inhibition, and cognition are involved in planning and executing a violent act. Any of these functions can be impaired or distorted by illness. Specifically, many different types of illnesses may give rise to agitation and aggressive behavior: psychiatric illnesses, neurological disorders such as dementia or frontal lobe damage, and many general medical disorders. However, some types of mental disorders are more likely than others to be associated with aggressive behavior. Some, such as antisocial personality disorder and intermittent explosive disorder, are by definition associated with aggression.

A particular violent act, regardless of the person's diagnosis, may or may not be related to psychopathology. Violence may be normal under certain circumstances (e.g., self-defense). Coercive or predatory violence, though antisocial, is often adaptive and rewarded.

Psychosis

All psychotic states may be associated with violence and agitation. Unplanned violence is often a result of agitation in disorganized psychotic patients and is therefore less focused and less dangerous. For example, a disorganized psychotic patient may respond to a bump, shove, or physical closeness as a homosexual threat and respond immediately. On the other hand, psychotic patients can have prominent, systematized delusional systems, which are typical of patients with paranoid schizophrenia or delusional disorder. Organized delusional systems often center on a specific person whom the patient sees as persecuting or depriving in some way—often a family member or someone well known to the patient. Because patients with paranoid schizophrenia retain many functions, they can organize their behavior in order to plan and carry out, using a weapon, a premeditated attack on their perceived persecutor. Among psychotic forensic patients, the more serious the violent act, the more delusions appear to have a direct role in the violent act (Taylor 1998).

Mania

Patients who are manic but not psychotic are more often angry and agitated than assaultive. Physical struggles may result when staff members attempt to contain manic patients with ambitious plans and psychomotor acceleration. Because of irritability, they may overreact to the behavior of other patients. Because their own behavior is often loud, active, intrusive, sexual, and belligerent, they can also provoke other patients, which can result in a fight.

Dementia

Dementia is very much associated with agitation. Nearly 50% of patients with dementia present with agitation some time during the course of their disorder (Tariot 1999). Patients with severe cognitive impairment are more likely to be agitated. Aggression in elderly patients with dementia is often reactive and impulsive. In a study of 20 elderly nursing home residents with dementia, only 18% of assaults were against other residents, usually in response to "uninvited advances," such as lying in the assailant's bed. Most assaults were on staff, and most of these occurred when staff interacted with patients in a physical way (e.g., during attempts to bathe or dress patients) (Bridges-Parlet et al. 1994).

Temporal Lobe Epilepsy

Aggressive behavior occurring during or immediately after a psychomotor seizure, when patients are confused, is generally purposeless, undirected, and rare. Like the aggression of demented patients, it is often provoked by staff attempts to physically interact with these individuals. Overall, the rate of violence resulting from temporal lobe epilepsy is exaggerated.

Head Trauma

Head trauma, particularly frontal lobe injury, is associated with irritability and assaultiveness. Often disinhibited, these patients have lost the ability to show restraint in provocative situations and react quickly and aggressively. Head trauma patients' usual coping strategies may be overwhelmed by a sudden change in their environment. Because their cognitive skills are limited, they may become agitated and aggressive. History, neurological symptoms, and electroencephalographic abnormalities pointing to head trauma all aid in the diagnostic process.

Pathophysiology

Although both agitation and aggression are not linked to specific diagnoses and have separate underlying pathophysiologies, these syndromes are pathophysiologically linked to the mechanisms responsible for the associated diagnostic presentation. In addition, both syndromes, agitation and aggression, overlap to a certain degree, both phenomenologically and pathophysiologically. Aggressive patients can be agitated and severe agitation can lead to aggressive behaviors. In this section, we review pathophysiology factors related to agitation and aggression.

Pathophysiology of Agitation

There is little literature on the underlying biological mechanisms of agitation as a separate and specific syndrome. Clues to specific underlying mechanisms are provided by the understanding of the mechanisms of the disorders that manifest with agitation. Specific neurotransmitter dysregulations are associated with these disorders and may be implicated in the pathophysiology of agitation (Table 4–1), as described later in this section (for a more extensive review, see Lindenmayer 2000).

Depression and Agitation

In agitated depression, both severity of depression and degree of anxiety tend to correlate closely with agitation. This results in three psychopathologically overlapping domains: depression, anxiety, and agitation. In terms of pathophysiology, there are probably two significant underlying mechanisms: 1) hyperactive hypothalamic-pituitary-adrenal (HPA) axis (HPA overactivity), and 2) increased serotonergic responsivity, as demonstrated by some abnormal responses to serotonergic challenges (Germine et al. 1992; Mintzer et al. 1998). Increased serotonergic transmission can trigger anxiety and agitation in vulnerable individuals. Other underlying neurotransmitter dysregulations have been postulated, such as decreased γ-aminobutyric acid (GABA)–ergic function and increased noradrenergic activity. In this situation, one would try to reduce the arousal through increasing GABAergic inhibition and decreasing noradrenergic transmission. Drugs, such

Table 4–1. Agitation in different clinical disorders: overview of underlying pathophysiological mechanisms

Agitated depression	Serotonergic, GABAergic, noradrenergic dysfunction
Mania	↑ Dopamine
Panic disorder and GAD	↑ Norepinephrine; ↓ GABA
Dementia	↓ GABA; serotonergic deficit; ↑ norepinephrine
Delirium	↓ GABA
Substance-induced agitation	Multiple causative mechanisms
Acute psychosis	↑ Dopamine
Aggression	↑ Dopamine; ↑ norepinephrine; ↓ serotonin; ↓ GABA

Note. ↑ = increase in levels; ↓ = decrease in levels. GABA = γ-aminobutyric acid; GAD = generalized anxiety disorder.

as GABAergic agonists (e.g., valproic acid, benzodiazepines), that increase GABAergic function and drugs that decrease noradrenergic transmission are helpful.

Dementia and Agitation

Three systems have been associated with agitation in dementia: GABAergic deficits, higher sensitivity to norepinephrine (Mintzer et al. 1998), and reduced serotonergic functions (Soininen et al. 1981). Interestingly, valproic acid, a GABAergic agonist, has been widely reported as an effective antiagitation and antiaggression agent in patients with dementia with agitation (Schatzberg and DeBattista 1999). Patients with higher sensitivity to norepinephrine might be candidates for intervention with dopamine antagonists. Dopamine antagonists with minimal liability regarding extrapyramidal side effects (EPS) (e.g., atypical antipsychotics) are indicated here. Other situations may call for serotonin$_{1A}$ (5-HT$_{1A}$) agonists to enhance serotonergic functioning.

Agitation and Psychosis

Agitation is often part of an acute psychotic episode and is phenomenologically related to the positive symptom domain. Dopaminergic pathways are the primary pathways implicated in the pathophysiology of positive symptoms, with serotonergic, GABA-ergic, and glutamatergic dysfunctions as secondary modulating mechanisms.

Acute psychotic states may represent a mesocortical disconnection syndrome resulting from limbic dopaminergic hyperactivity with an interruption of glutamatergic modulation of dopaminergic neurotransmission and reduced GABAergic inhibition. This may lead to reduced prefrontal cortical activity and positive, negative, and cognitive symptoms. Dysfunctions in serotonergic pathways have also been implicated in the pathophysiology of psychosis. Serotonin$_{2A}$ (5-HT$_{2A}$) pathways modulate nigrostriatal dopaminergic activity, which may explain why 5-HT$_{2A}$ antagonism increases dopamine neurotransmission. This mechanism may underlie the beneficial effects of atypical antipsychotics on extrapyramidal symptoms; these compounds all show pronounced 5-HT$_{2A}$ affinity. These drugs also reach high occupancy rates of cortical 5-HT$_{2A}$ receptors, which may relate to their beneficial effects on negative symptoms. However, for the purpose of treating positive symptoms in the emergency setting, rapid and effective dopamine$_2$ (D$_2$) antagonism is crucial. Additional sedating quality, conferred by high histamine$_1$ (H$_1$) affinity, may also be desirable. Atypical compounds in use at present, such as risperidone, olanzapine, quetiapine, and clozapine, possess some of the characteristics listed above. Another advantage of atypical agents may be the observation that D$_2$ receptor antagonism occurs primarily in the limbic system, which is the target area for positive symptoms, rather than in cortical areas. Although typical antipsychotics deliver appropriate D$_2$ antagonism, they may not be ideal antiagitation compounds, because they are all associated with significant EPS.

Akathisia induced by treatment with antipsychotics can be confused with agitation. The clinical description of akathisia includes difficulty sitting still, repetitive leg movements, restlessness, subjective feeling of inner agitation, and overall irregular movements. Akathisia is thought to be related to nigrostriatal dopamine blockade induced by D$_2$ antagonism. In addition, increased central norepinephrine may antagonize mesocortical dopamine function even further. Atypical antipsychotics are particularly associated with akathisia, which can occur early in treatment. Interventions consist of reducing nigrostriatal dopamine blockade by reducing the dose of the antipsychotic drug or by introducing a β-adrenergic blocker to reduce the central norepinephrine hyperactivity. In addition, an increase in GABAergic inhibition, through use of benzodiazepines, is another way of treating akathisia.

Pathophysiology of Aggressive Behavior

Multiple factors and mechanisms are involved in the development of aggressive behavior and interact in a complex fashion. Aggressive behavior is not linked with any one specific diagnosis but, rather, is the result of complex interactions among environmental, genetic, and biological factors.

Biological Factors

Biological factors include congenital, demographic, neurological, neurocognitive, and neurochemical factors (for review, see Volavka 1995). Genetics offers some insight into our understanding of impulsive aggression. Both twin and adoption studies suggest a partial heritable basis for impulsive aggression (Bohman et al. 1982; Coccaro et al. 1989). Nielsen et al. (1994) found an association between the L-tryptophan hydroxylase (L-TPH) allele and reduced cerebrospinal fluid (CSF) 5-hydroxyindoleacetic acid (5-HIAA) concentration in impulsive offenders and nonoffenders with suicide attempts. Male personality disorder patients homozygous for the L-TPH allele had higher scores on irritability and aggression measures (New et al. 1998). Hallikainen et al. (1999) found an association of low-activity serotonin transporter (5-HTT) promoter genotype and early-onset alcoholism with habitual impulsive behavior. It appears, then, that certain alleles in serotonin-related genes may confer greater vulnerability to impulsive aggression to certain individuals.

The role of gender in violence is of interest to our society, where arrest rates, victimization surveys, and self-reports show a preponderance of male perpetrators. Males are often implicated, particularly in serious violent offenses. While rearing factors may significantly contribute to this gender gap, biological factors may also play a key role. For example, males are more vulnerable to the aggression-mediating effects of low serotonergic and central norepinephrine hyperactivity (Brown et al. 1979; Lamprecht et al. 1972). Males are more likely to develop alcoholism, a disease with some biological etiology and strong associations with aggression (Bushman and Cooper 1990).

Neurological Correlates of Violence

The neurology of violence has been studied extensively. Multiple nonspecific neurological impairments have been found in patients with histories of violence (Convit et al. 1988). McKinlay et al. (1981) reported that nearly 70% of patients with head injuries exhibit irritability and aggression. This may account for some of the neuropsychological, neurological, and electroencephalographic abnormalities found in violent subjects (see Volavka 1995, pp. 97–98). Specifically, lesions on the orbitomedial area of the frontal lobe are associated with impulsive and hostile behavior (Blumer and Benson 1975; Grafman et al. 1996). Heinrichs (1989) found that frontal brain lesions were related to documented violent incidents in 45 neuropsychiatric inpatients. Highly violent tendencies have also been associated with computed tomography (CT) scan and electroencephalographic abnormalities in the temporal lobes (Wong et al. 1994). However, most studies supporting correlations among violence and temporal lobe lesions have not been well controlled.

Research has shown that electroencephalographic abnormalities correlate with violent behavior. Qualitative electroencephalographic assessments show abnormalities in 57% of persistently violent offenders versus 12% of offenders who committed an isolated violent act (Williams 1969). There are no specific areas of the brain where electroencephalographic abnormalities are consistently present; however, many abnormalities are located in frontotemporal areas. In addition, quantitative assessments show an association between electroencephalographic slowing and violence. Raine et al. (1998), using positron emission tomography (PET) imaging, found that affective murderers had lower left and right prefrontal functioning than did nonviolent control subjects. This supports the hypothesis that emotional, impulsive violent offenders are less able to regulate impulse control because of deficient prefrontal drive regulation.

Neuropsychology sheds more light on aggressive behavior. Neuropsychological test batteries show associations between violence and multiple functional brain impairments. Yeudall (1977) compared 25 aggressive psychopathic patients with 25 depressed criminal patients. Neurological impairments for both cohorts were found in the anterior regions of the brain; however, impairments in the aggressive group were more frequently lateralized to the dominant hemisphere. Patients with histories of violence generally show impaired performance on tests of cognitive, perceptual, and psychomotor abilities (Moffitt and Silva 1988; Spellacy 1978).

Low intelligence has been linked to crime independently of socioeconomic status, avoidance of apprehension, and sampling bias (Hirschi and Hindelang 1977; Hodgins 1992). Low full-scale IQ scores have been linked with violent crime in some reports (Kahn 1959; Langevin et al. 1987; Spellacy 1978); however, others have found no difference in IQ between violent and nonviolent offenders (Yeudall 1977). Furthermore, the effects of mediating variables, such as antisocial personality disorder or impulsiveness, remain unclear.

Neurochemistry

Certain dysfunctions in neurotransmitter and hormonal functioning—for example, insulin (Virkkunen 1986) and testosterone (Dabbs et al. 1995)—are associated with violent behavior.

Norepinephrine. Noradrenergic hyperactivity correlates highly with aggressive behavior (Gerra et al. 1997). Träskman-Bendz et al. (1992) found elevated CSF 3-methoxy-4-hydroxyphenylglycol (MHPG) levels in violent suicide attempters compared with nonviolent suicide attempters. Increased β-adrenergic receptor binding sites in prefrontal and temporal areas have been found more commonly in violent suicide victims than in accident victims (Mann et al. 1986).

Two enzymes metabolize norepinephrine: monoamine oxidase (the isoenzymes A and B ; MAO-A, MAO-B) and catechol-O-methyltransferase (COMT). Belfrage et al. (1992) found low MAO activity in platelets of violent offenders. Cases et al. (1995) found that male "knock-out" mice lacking the MAO-A gene show more aggressive behavior than those with normal genetic makeup. Poor metabolism of norepinephrine leads to hyperarousal of the noradrenergic system and thus possibly to aggressive behavior. COMT polymorphism normally results in three- to fourfold variation in enzymatic activity. The presence of the allele for the less active form of the enzyme has been found to be associated with violent behavior in schizophrenic and schizoaffective patients, predominantly in males (Lachman et al. 1998; Strous et al. 1997). Male knock-out mice deficient in the COMT gene also showed aggressive behavior (Gogos et al. 1998). Both observations support the role of noradrenergic hyperactivity in the pathophysiology of violence. This may explain the beneficial therapeutic effects of β-blockers in reducing aggressive behaviors in chronic psychiatric inpatients (Ratey et al. 1992).

Serotonin. An understanding of central serotonergic functioning is key to understanding the role of serotonin in aggressive behavior. CSF 5-HIAA levels reflect presynaptic serotonergic activity in the brain. Reduced levels of 5-HIAA indicate a reduction in central serotonin (5-HT) activity. Prevailing research indicates that low CSF 5-HIAA levels are related to impulsivity but not specifically to violence. When a 5-HT receptor agonist such as fenfluramine is introduced, presynaptic stores of 5-HT are released and postsynaptic 5-HT receptors are stimulated with inhibition of 5-HT reuptake. Using the fenfluramine challenge paradigm, Coccaro (1989) found that prolactin response was reduced in men with personality disorders associated with aggression—a finding supporting a central serotonergic deficit. In addition, low CSF 5-HIAA values have been found in depressive patients with a history of violent suicide attempts (Åsberg et al. 1976). Linnoila et al. (1983) identified low CSF 5-HIAA levels in Finnish murderers with an alcohol abuse history who were classified as impulsive. In another study, low CSF 5-HIAA levels were noted in 20 male arsonists who set fires impulsively (Virkkunen et al. 1987).

However, data from other samples have shown either no correlation or a positive correlation between CSF 5-HIAA levels and aggression. Coccaro (1992) found no significant correlation between CSF 5-HIAA levels and life history or self-reported aggression measures in adult male veterans with personality disorders. High CSF 5-HIAA levels were related to aggression in normal adult subjects (Castellanos et al. 1994) and in children with disruptive behavioral disorders (Moller et al. 1996).

Gamma-aminobutyric acid.   Potentiation of central GABAergic activity is associated with decreased predatory aggression. Conversely, decreased GABAergic activity predicts increased aggression (Haug et al. 1980; Puglisi-Allegra 1980; Simler et al. 1983). Support for a role of decreased central GABAergic activity comes also from certain therapeutic interventions. Benzodiazepines have been reported to reduce aggression in various studies (Christmas and Maxwell 1970; Randall et al. 1960; Valzelli 1973). Valproate also has well-documented antiaggressive effects, which have been documented in patients with bipolar disorder, dementia, and schizophrenia (for review, see Lindenmayer and Kotsaftis 2000).

Assessment Issues

Agitation

Emergency room psychiatric patients who present with agitation and aggression can be the most challenging patients. The evaluation of such patients is often limited by the lack of a full history. The patient may be unable or unwilling to give a coherent history, and family or friends may not be available. The mental status examination may also be incomplete because of the lack of cooperation or the patient's level of psychosis.

An important early diagnostic decision is to determine whether the acute agitation is due to an underlying organic state or to a functional state. Findings that should raise the index of suspicion for an organic underlying cause are a very acute onset of symptoms, fluctuating levels of consciousness, disorientation to time and place, short-term memory difficulties, concurrent medical illness with physical findings, and a history free of previous psychiatric episodes. Possible organic causes for agitation should be excluded; they include hyperthyroidism, hypoglycemia, cerebral hypoxia due to cardiac or pulmonary dysfunctions, withdrawal states from alcohol and narcotics, and acute intoxication with substances of abuse (see Chapter 2, this volume).

Functional states giving rise to agitation can be seen with anxious depressions or acute schizophrenic episodes. In the latter situation, other evidence of schizophrenia, such as auditory or visual hallucinations, irrational thinking, and inappropriate affect, should be sought. Acute manic states may also be accompanied by agitation. Usually, the manic patient's expansiveness, euphoric mood, and grandiose ideas will help in the differential diagnosis. An acute, nonpsychotic anxiety state can give rise to agitation with either fixed anxiety, centered on a particular situation, or free-floating anxiety. Symptoms reported by patients may include feelings of panic or impending danger, restlessness, hyperactivity, tremor, perspiration, dry mouth, tachycardia, and possibly hyperventilation.

Violence Risk Assessment

Mental health professionals assess an individual's potential risk of harm to others on an ongoing basis in outpatient practice; in emergency rooms, when they decide to admit or not to admit; and in hospitals, when they decide to release or retain patients. These are very important decisions, because they affect the physical safety of other human beings and because those who make them may be held accountable for their outcome.

Decisions to admit, release, or retain should be well informed and well considered. Difficult decisions should be confirmed by a second opinion and documented with a specific risk assessment. A careful consideration of risk factors during the assessment will help in the prediction of violence for the particular patient. The assessment should include collection of relevant data, consideration of the data, acknowledgment of potential risks, and provision for adequate community support and safeguards. Specific environmental risk factors that may contribute to reemergence of aggressive behavior need to be identified. For the assessment of patients' safe functioning in the community, the clinician must review patients' environment and predicted symptomatology in the community.

Patient-Related Risk Factors

The assessment of the risk an individual patient poses in the community may benefit from knowledge of actuarial prediction or the factors that are related to violence in large groups of adult patients in the community. Some factors, such as patient traits and history, are unmodifiable, whereas others are modifiable (e.g., state [e.g., psychosis] and environmental factors).

Traits particularly relevant to violence prediction are sex, age, and socioeconomic status. Male sex, youth, and relative poverty predict violent crime in the general population. Among adults with mental illness, youth is associated with arrests for violent crime among male civil inpatients released into the community (Klassen and O'Connor 1998). College graduates, whether mentally ill or not, were rarely violent in Stueve and Link's (1997) study of young Israelis.

The role of sex, an unmodifiable trait, is more complex. Clinicians often underestimate the potential for violence among women (Lidz et al. 1993). Women with mental illness, as well as women in the general population, seem less likely to be arrested (Monahan et al. 2001, p. 43) or convicted for violent crime (Wessely 1998). Some investigators find female assaults less severe and less likely to cause injuries (Monahan et al. 2001, p. 43); others disagree (Newhill et al. 1995). In the MacArthur study, aggression among women consisted mainly of pushing, slapping, shoving, and throwing objects, whereas violence among men consisted of kicking, biting, and hitting. Women were at least as likely as men to be physically aggressive during the year after they were discharged from the hospital (Monahan et al. 2001, p. 41). Newhill and colleagues (1995) also concluded that sex was not a strong predictor of violence. In their sample, violent mentally ill women were more likely to be depressed than violent mentally ill men. The men, however, were more likely to have a primary diagnosis of substance abuse (Newhill et al. 1995). Mentally ill women are more likely than mentally ill men to be violent at home, and their targets are more likely to be family members (Monahan et al. 2001, pp. 41–43; Newhill et al. 1995).

Historical Risk Factors

Historical factors are strong predictors of aggressive behavior. As clinicians know well, past behavior predicts future behavior. Past arrests for violent crime predict future arrests. In a London study of a large group of adults with schizophrenia (Wessely 1998), the strongest predictor of conviction for a crime was a conviction before the onset of illness. Substance abuse history and diagnosis of conduct disorder during childhood are also useful predictors. Another measure of early psychopathology, the age at onset of mental illness, also predicts conviction for crime. Wessely (1998) found that the earlier the age at onset of mental illness, the greater the risk of acquiring a criminal record.

Antisocial personality and substance abuse are stronger predictors of aggression than are psychotic symptoms. However, active psychotic symptoms, particularly command auditory hallucinations to hurt others, add significantly to risk. Suspiciousness, anger, and thoughts of hurting others also add to risk. The presence of hallucinations and comorbidity with substance abuse increase the risk of violence for all adults with major mental illness, including those with schizophrenia. The risk seems to be additive rather than multiplicative—that is, the risk of substance abuse is added to the independent risk of major mental illness (for review, see Eronen et al. 1998). Finally, psychotropic medication noncompliance predicts violence (Swartz et al. 1998).

Environmental Risk Factors

The clinician should also consider the patient's environment when making a risk assessment. With whom will the patient be living? In what neighborhood? In the MacArthur study (Silver et al. 1999), patients discharged to neighborhoods with high levels of poverty were more likely to be violent than those discharged to more advantaged neighborhoods. These results remained after other salient traits, such as age, substance abuse, and socioeconomic status, were controlled for. The victims of violence perpe-trated by adults with mental illness are most often people they know, usually family members. In contrast, victims of violence committed by the general public are more often strangers. In a study of violent behavior of discharged psychiatric patients with schizophrenia or major affective disorder (Estroff et al. 1998), 84% of the targets were familiar with their assailant; 30% were immediate family members. Mothers of patients were the single largest group of victims. Other significant predictors of victim-ization were residing with the patient, being the patient's source of financial support, and hostility toward the patient. This data set suggests that aggression in persons with mental illness arises out of long-standing resentment and interpersonal conflict.

Risk Assessment in the Interview

The clinician should also learn how the patient understands his or her previous violent behavior. Can the patient make a con-nection between intoxication or treatment noncompliance and previous violence? How able is the patient to change old habits? Supervised medication administration or substance abuse treat-ment may be necessary to decrease a patient's risk in the commu-nity. The clinician should also learn if the patient has a regular, identifiable target and, if so, contact the target. Prudent planning dictates that the patient and target live separately.

A careful risk assessment should include documentation of the patient's traits and history that may be predictors of future violence. The assessment should contain an exploration of the circumstances of the violence, the target, and the patient's state and the environment during episodes of violence. Traits and his-tory are unmodifiable, but psychopathology and state of intoxi-cation are modifiable.

Treatment

Settings

Treatment issues of patients who present with acute agitation and aggression will be very much influenced by the setting in which they present. Whereas the diagnosis of a patient with agitation or an acute assaultive episode in an inpatient setting will usually be well known, this information is usually missing in patients newly presenting to the emergency room. The setting will also determine the type and availability of acute treatments, of trained staff, and of specialized rooms and equipment to deal with the emergency competently. The final disposition of the emergency will be significantly affected by the setting. A brief description of these issues is presented below.

The Emergency Service

Important factors to consider in the emergency room setting are the patient's expectations about the kind of help he or she will receive. These expectations may in part determine the presenting agitated or assaultive behaviors. A patient who is seeking hospital admission at all cost will at times resort to dramatic displays in order to gain admission. The family's expectations must also be considered, because they are the ones who may have defined the emergency to begin with and determined the need to bring the patient to the emergency room.

The emergency service should provide a quiet space where the agitated or violent patient can be isolated and a sense of crowding can be prevented. If appropriate, the examiner will inquire about weapons. If the patient has a weapon, the interviewer should refuse to examine the patient until the weapon is surrendered to him or her or to security guards. If the patient is not in restraints, it is important that he or she have enough space to move without disrupting other ongoing activities. Restraints can be removed only when there is evidence that the patient is in control of the aggressive impulses or the agitation. Ventilation and talking down techniques can be used with or without parenteral medication effectively in this setting. The most important step in the emergency room evaluation of an assaultive or agitated patient is to help the patient bring his or her agitation and violence rapidly under control.

The Inpatient Setting

Agitated or assaultive episodes usually occur during the first few days of an inpatient admission and are often seen in the context of acute psychosis. At that point, the patient may be better known to the staff and diagnostic considerations may have been sufficiently clarified to allow specific treatment of the underlying cause of agitation or assaultiveness. Possible treatment interventions include talking down, which is the preferred mode; time out in a quiet room; an oral or parenteral medication for agitation; seclusion; and, in extreme cases, physical restraints. It is important, once a violent episode has happened and has been brought under control, to have a debriefing meeting with the staff and later with the patient, to gain better insight into the precipitating events and to develop early prevention techniques.

Assaultive episodes that occur later in the hospitalization, after the acute phase, may indicate that the ongoing treatment regimen is not fully effective or that the patient is undergoing an incipient relapse. These episodes need to be reviewed with an aim of addressing any needed change in the current treatment.

Behavioral Treatments

Initial Steps

Highly agitated patients often arrive at the emergency room with friends or family. A rapid judgment must be made as to whether the companions are contributing to the problem or to its solution. If the patient feels more secure with those accompanying him or her, they should be present during the interview. However, it is wise under these circumstances to ask the patient whether it is permissible to discuss personal matters freely. This should also be noted in the chart. During the interview, the examiner should be active and indicate that something will be done to relieve the acute agitation. Once the patient is sufficiently communicative and rapport has been established, a careful history should be taken in order to document the circumstances associated with the emergence of agitation. There should be an inquiry into precipitating events, for situations that worsen or improve the agitation, and for other symptoms associated with the agitation. This inquiry will also serve therapeutic purposes, since it allows the patient to ventilate some of the feelings underlying the agitation, so that the patient can use the reality testing of the interventions to reorganize his or her usual coping mechanisms (see Chapter 5, this volume).

It is essential to understand that although those around the patient are frightened by the assaultiveness, the patient who perceives himself or herself out of control is even more so. Any delay or half-hearted attempt to control the patient's violence, therefore, will result in even more violence, since the patient realizes that the clinician is unable to control him or her. An agitated patient who has not lost control may respond to a calm and nonthreatening verbal intervention. However, if the patient is severely agitated and psychotic or delirious, more immediate pharmacological treatment with an antipsychotic or benzodiazepine will first have to be instituted. If the patient already is restrained and sitting in a wheelchair, the physician should conduct the initial assessment under these conditions until the physician is completely sure that the patient is in control of his or her impulses. The patient should be asked directly by the physician about this; in particular, the patient should be told to indicate whether he feels that he is about to become aggressive again.

Patients who have not yet lost control but who seem to be on the verge of doing so should be approached in a calm but firm manner. Here again, the physician should keep in mind the need to protect both himself or herself and the patient. The door of the room should be kept open to reduce the patient's possible feeling of being trapped. There should be trained personnel nearby to help restrain the patient if violence erupts.

Verbal Techniques

Verbal communication with the patients can be made only with patients who have not yet lost control. Such communication should be made in a clear, firm fashion from the start and should be directed at two main points. First, it should aim at exploring the cause of the patient's loss of control and of his or her ensuing rage. Second, if the patient is confused about his or her present environment or disoriented, this should be addressed by indicating repeatedly where he or she is, the purpose of the examination, and the identity of the people attending to him or her at the moment. Throughout the interview, care should be taken to explain every procedure or action in order to minimize any possible misinterpretation by the patient.

Communication with paranoid patients presents special problems, since usually they have been brought for treatment against their will and do not consider themselves to be sick. The patient's position is characterized by suspiciousness, mistrust, and anger. Development of rapport with the patient requires that his or her distrust and resentment be recognized and addressed; for example, the physician can acknowledge that the patient was brought against his will. The patient then may go into a long tirade about the harmful things his family is doing to him. The physician should permit the patient to give his account; in particular, he should abstain from challenging the delusional state, since it would be provocative. It is more important to ask the patient the reasons for his being the focus of his perceived persecutions. If the patient directly asks the interviewer to agree with his delusions, the latter should respond that he can understand the interpretation of the facts by the patient but that his own interpretation might be different.

Once communication with the patient is established and some of the factors that brought on the loss of control are discussed, a more detailed history usually can be gathered. This history should be compared with the history given by the family, which may differ significantly. In particular, patients may want to minimize past violent behavior and psychopathology, since it is difficult for them to see themselves as sick.

During the interview, a careful mental status examination should be performed. If the patient is calm enough to tolerate a physical examination, this should also be done.

Quiet Room/Time Out

If a patient has not yet lost control and is cooperative, an opportunity for "time out" in a quiet room, if available, can be provided. This area has to have open access and must be under close staff supervision. It offers the patient a time away from stimulation, an opportunity for reconstituting after an agitated blow up, or a place to experience painful emotions. This type of isolation should not be confused with seclusion, as it is voluntary and unlocked. The room should have few furnishings and no hazardous objects.

Physical Restraint and Seclusion

If verbal techniques and pharmacological interventions have been used but have not succeeded in effectively treating the aggressive or violent episode, staff may have to resort to physical restraints or seclusion. These are procedures that both staff and patients usually find unpleasant; they are clearly high-risk procedures that can lead, if not done properly, to injury and psychological trauma. They should be undertaken only by well-trained staff who are accustomed to working together as a team and have trained together. The overall principle governing seclusion and restraint is to use the least restrictive alternative available to treat the episode.

Although most psychiatric staff will see a clear rationale and indication for effective physical containment techniques, these techniques have of late been intensely scrutinized by regulatory bodies. The latest Joint Commission on Accreditation of Healthcare Organizations (JCAHO) recommendations (2002) describe these procedures as "aversive experience with potential for serious physical and emotional consequences including death. Organizations are required to continually explore ways to decrease and eliminate use through training, leadership commitment and performance improvement." The specific definitions by JCAHO standards are as follows:

> *Restraint:* Direct application of physical force to a patient, with or without the patient's permission, to restrict his or her freedom of movement. The physical force may be human, mechanical devices, or a combination thereof.
> *Seclusion:* Involuntary confinement of a person alone in a locked room. The behavioral health care reasons for the use of restraint or seclusion are primarily to protect the patient against injury to self or others because of an emotional or behavioral disorder. (JCAHO 2002, p. 123)

The regulations emphasize that nonphysical interventions are always preferred and that restraints are always the last resort.

The Centers for Medicare and Medicaid Services (CMS) Hospital Conditions of Participation for Patients' Rights specify that "use of restraint must be selected only when other less restrictive measures have been found to be ineffective to protect the patient or others from harm" (Centers for Medicare and Medicaid Services 1999). This reduced emphasis on the therapeutic benefits of restraints is thought by some to be a consequence of instances of abuse, medical complications, and death in the context of applying these techniques. It is therefore crucial that staff be well trained in these techniques, comfortable using them, and fully knowledgeable in the local regulatory requirements and documentation.

Procedure.   The restraint process basically involves three different sets of interventions. First, someone makes the decision to initiate restraints. Then, a group of staff members physically places the patient in restraints. Finally, a face-to-face assessment is done to evaluate the need for restraints. The CMS Hospital Conditions of Participation for Patients' Rights indicate that "the use of restraint or seclusion must be in accordance with the order of a physician or other licensed independent practitioner permitted by the State and hospital to order seclusion or restraint" (Centers for Medicare and Medicaid Services 1999). Seclusion can be initiated by nursing staff, but it has to be ordered within 1 hour by a physician. The physician or other licensed independent practitioner must conduct a face-to-face examination of the patient within 1 hour, which includes a review of the patient's physical and psychological state. The initial order for seclusion or restraints can only have a maximum duration of 4 hours, after which the patient has to be reevaluated by the physician and a new order has to be written. For patients under 18 years of age, this duration is reduced to 2 hours. The CMS interim final rules specify continuous audio and visual monitoring while in restraints. The JCAHO regulations specify continuous in-person monitoring for individuals in restraints (with continuous audiovisual monitoring allowed after the first hour for patients in seclusion). Staff is required to conduct 15-minute checks to assess vital signs, any signs of injury, the patient's psychological state, and readiness to discontinue seclusion or restraints.

In physically restraining patients or bringing an agitated and uncooperative patient into seclusion, it is important that the staff work as a team and that enough staff members be present both to demonstrate nonnegotiable force to the patient and to perform the procedure in a safe manner. Team members need to remove dangerous objects from their persons. The team needs to have a leader who assigns the task of holding a particular part of the patient to each team member. Each extremity is held by one team member, and a fifth person is assigned to hold the patient's head in order to prevent any possible injury to staff and patient alike. Only when restraint is successful can any pharmacological agent be given. Debriefing of staff is also important to ascertain any trauma to staff as a result of the intervention and to provide support after a serious violent incident.

Documentation. Complete documentation is crucial for seclusion-and-restraint episodes. Clinicians need to follow the applicable local regulations, which typically include documentation of the physician's order for seclusion or type of restraint with date, time, allowable duration, and signature, together with reason for the intervention; prior and alternative interventions; notification of family; documentation of 15-minute checks; evidence of physical and psychological assessment by the physician; record of medications administered with their effects; and criteria for termination of the intervention. A debriefing note needs to be added that documents precipitants to the incident and alternative treatments, modifications of the treatment plan, and the patient's psychological and physical well-being after the intervention.

Pharmacotherapy

Patients who are agitated and potentially violent will often require pharmacological interventions. Principles of treatment are 1) rapid onset of action, 2) easy medication administration, 3) minimal side effects, and 4) minimal pharmacokinetic interactions with other currently used medications or possible underlying medical conditions. The medications most frequently used in this context are antipsychotics and benzodiazepines.

The two initial questions to be decided are the choice of medication and the route of administration. The choice of medication should, whenever possible, be guided by the underlying diagnosis. Psychotic agitation should be treated with an antipsychotic up to the maximum daily dose generally employed, while an agitated panic state will best respond to a benzodiazepine. Often, however, the diagnosis of the underlying state will not be clear yet and treatment will have to proceed along syndromal lines. When no data on the possible underlying diagnosis are available, a benzodiazepine is the favored approach.

The question of route of administration may be strongly influenced by the level of the patient's cooperation. The major advantage of the intramuscular route is its use in involuntary treatment. Other therapeutic differences between the oral and intramuscular routes are relatively minor (Allen 2000). In a study comparing oral risperidone concentrate and lorazepam with intramuscular haloperidol and lorazepam, Currier (2000) found that most agitated patients assented to oral medication. In a survey of 51 emergency services, medical directors estimated that only 1 of 10 emergency patients requires an injection (Currier and Allen 1999). Clearly, the use of oral medications for agitated or aggressive patients may be a realistic option in the emergency setting.

Although intravenous administration shows the fastest onset of action, it is rarely feasible in the emergency situation. The onset of intramuscular haloperidol is usually from 30 to 60 minutes. Intramuscular absorption of lorazepam and midazolam is also rapid, between 15 and 30 minutes. Clonazepam administered intramuscularly appears to be slower in onset than haloperidol, as reported in manic patients (Chouinard et al. 1993).

Whenever possible, these medication strategies should be discussed with patients to obtain their consent. For patients who are expected to become agitated or violent over the course of their illness, a treatment preference contract should be worked out as an advance directive between the patient and the mental health team. This will involve the patient in his or her care and help the physician to better determine the best-suited medication and/or behavioral interventions in case of agitation or violence.

In case of involuntary medication administration, care has to be taken that the treatment indication is well documented and that the applicable mental hygiene regulations regarding the duration of treatment and the required medical supervision are followed.

Antipsychotics

Typical antipsychotics.   The choice here is between a high-potency compound (e.g., haloperidol), which is less sedating, and a sedating low-potency antipsychotic (e.g., chlorpromazine). The advantages and disadvantages for each are outlined in Table 4–2. Clearly, for agitation and aggression seen in the emergency service, a high-potency compound is preferable, because such compounds tend to have fewer cardiovascular side effects.

Table 4–2.   Low-potency versus high-potency antipsychotic side effects

Low-potency	Hypotensive
	Lowers seizure threshold
	Sedating
	Lower EPS risk
	More anticholinergic side effects
High-potency	Nonsedating
	Few cardiovascular effects
	Less anticholinergic
	High EPS risk
	Akathisia
	Neuroleptic malignant syndrome

Note.   EPS = extrapyramidal side effects.

Akathisia is a particularly problematic phenomenon with high-potency drugs, because this subjective sense of restlessness often cannot be distinguished from agitated anxiety. A frequent practice is to combine a high-potency antipsychotic with a short-acting benzodiazepine (e.g., lorazepam). This adjunctive treatment offers sedation and treatment for possible acute EPS (e.g., acute dystonic reaction) and may also be effective in treating akathisia. Often, an anticholinergic may have to be added later on for the treatment of EPS. On the other hand, low-potency drugs do not require additional sedative treatments and present a lesser risk for EPS because of their anticholinergic profile, but they may induce significant hypotension in some patients.

A significant advantage of the typical antipsychotics is their availability in intramuscular form, which makes them still, despite the introduction of newer atypical drugs, the medications of choice in the present context. Rapid neuroleptization, which was at one time favored by physicians treating acutely psychotic patients who also were agitated, is no longer advisable. The onset of action and effectiveness are not superior to those of traditional dosage techniques (Donlon et al. 1980). Another adverse effect with typical antipsychotics, neuroleptic malignant syndrome (NMS), is of particular concern in patients with acute agitation who may become dehydrated. NMS occurs with a frequency of about 1%.

Another compound used specifically in the treatment of severe agitation in emergency settings is droperidol, which is available only in a parenteral formulation. However, because of its potential for QT_C prolongation and torsades de pointe, it has lost all its attractiveness.

Recommended dosages for acutely agitated psychotic patients are as follows: haloperidol 2–5 mg im every 1–4 hours together with lorazepam 2 mg im; or chlorpromazine 25–50 mg im every 1–4 hours. An alternative form of administration for haloperidol or chlorpromazine is the oral concentrate formulation mixed in orange juice, which is at times more acceptable to patients. An important principle of treatment with antipsychotics is to use the lowest effective dose in order to prevent unwanted side effects.

In case of agitation and violence in the context of drug withdrawal from sedative-hypnotics, antipsychotics are contraindicated because they lower the seizure threshold. Benzodiazepines are the treatment of choice in these situations.

High-potency antipsychotics are preferable to low-potency compounds in the treatment of agitation and violence in patients with delirium. Low-potency antipsychotics, because of their sedating and anticholinergic properties, may worsen the delirious states in these patients. Dosages of antipsychotics need to be adjusted in situations with elderly patients or with patients with cerebrovascular problems: haloperidol 0.5–2 mg im every 30 minutes to 1 hour can be given until the patient is calm.

Atypical antipsychotics. Atypical (or second-generation) antipsychotics are clearly superior to typical agents in terms of their lesser propensity for EPS and more beneficial profiles regarding other side effects. However, at this time, there is no intramuscular, short-acting form available, although an intramuscular form of olanzapine and ziprasidone may soon be available (Meehan et al. 2001). Having an intramuscular form of an atypical compound will make the process of switching to the oral form for longer-term treatment easier. There are two administration forms of atypical compounds that may be useful for emergency situations: a liquid risperidone form and a rapidly dissolving oral olanzapine form.

Benzodiazepines

Short-acting benzodiazepines (lorazepam or midazolam) are extremely helpful in the acute management of agitation and aggressive behavior. On the basis of a double-blind study comparing lorazepam 2 mg im and haloperidol 5 mg im as a prn medication for the control of assaultive or aggressive behavior, Salzman et al. (1991) found that both compounds were equally effective in controlling aggressive and psychotic symptoms but that patients on haloperidol had significantly more EPS. More recently, Battaglia et al. (1997) compared the acute antiagitation effects of either haloperidol and lorazepam alone with those of the combination of haloperidol and lorazepam. They found that the combination treatment was more effective than either treatment alone. In terms of benzodiazepines, lorazepam may be particularly useful because of its short half-life and the availability of intramuscular, intravenous, and oral forms. Given that haloperidol can cause significant EPS and can worsen phencyclidine intoxication, it is generally preferable to use parenteral lorazepam in many emergency situations. The usual dose for lorazepam is 2 mg im every 1–2 hours as needed. Other benzodiazepines whose use has been reported in patients with agitation and aggression are reviewed by Allen (2000). Flunitrazepam 1 mg has been found to be superior to haloperidol 5 mg on the Overt Aggression Scale (Dorevitch et al. 1999). Midazolam 5 mg has been reported to be superior to haloperidol 10 mg on a measure of motor agitation (Wyant et al. 1990).

Benzodiazepines have an excellent safety record compared with neuroleptics. The phenomenon of disinhibition is rare and only anecdotal. Worsening has not been noted in acute trials in emergency settings (Citrome and Volavka 1999). Another concern with benzodiazepines is respiratory depression in the context of alcohol or other sedative intoxication. There is a particular concern with midazolam use in emergency situations because of its association with respiratory depression and cardiac arrest when used in combination with an opioid (Nordt and Clark 1997).

Barbiturates

Safe and effective benzodiazepines have displaced barbiturates in the treatment of acute agitation and aggression. Barbiturates also have a high potential for abuse and dependence and are therefore less favored. However, in patients who do not respond to benzodiazepines, they still can be useful. Compounds with a shorter half-life, such as sodium amobarbital 250 mg im every 4 hours, would be preferable in order to avoid accumulation of the drug over time.

Other Medications

Less frequently used compounds are chloral hydrate and diphenhydramine. The latter is an antihistamine and has sedative properties. These drugs may be indicated in situations with patients who are prone to abuse sedative-hypnotic medications.

Conclusion

The relatively limited goal in a behavioral emergency with a patient with agitation or aggression is the termination of the emergency and the resumption or initiation of a more typical

---

therapeutic relationship with a focus on more active participation by the patient and a positive long-term outcome. Treatments offered during an emergency span the entire behavioral-pharmacological spectrum. After a full initial assessment of underlying psychiatric and medical causes, verbal interventions should attempt to establish contact with the patient in order to create a safe inner and outer environment. Pharmacological interventions should be short-term and directed at relieving anxious agitation, psychotic impulsivity, and loss of control. Behavioral interventions may have to be used if the preceding treatments fail or are refused. Whenever possible, patients should be involved in making choices in these different treatment approaches. During an emergency, the emphasis is on reestablishing inner and outer controls for the patient in the least coercive way.

References

Allen MH: Managing the agitated psychotic patient: a reappraisal of the evidence. J Clin Psychiatry 61 (suppl 14):11–20, 2000

Åsberg M, Träskman L, Thorén P: 5-HIAA in the cerebrospinal fluid: a biochemical suicide predictor? Arch Gen Psychiatry 33:1193–1197, 1976

Battaglia J, Moss S, Rush J, et al: Haloperidol, lorazepam, or both for psychotic agitation? A multicenter, prospective, double-blind, emergency department study. Am J Emerg Med 15(4):335–340, 1997

Belfrage H, Lidbert L, Oreland L: Platelet monoamine oxidase activity in mentally disordered violent offenders. Acta Psychiatr Scand 85(3): 218–221, 1992

Blumer D, Benson DF: Personality changes with frontal and temporal lobe lesions, in Psychiatric Aspects of Neurologic Disease. Edited by Benson DF, Blumer D. New York, Grune & Stratton, 1975, pp 151–170

Bohman M, Cloninger CR, Sigvardsson S, et al: Predisposition to petty criminality in Swedish adoptees, I: genetic and environmental heterogeneity. Arch Gen Psychiatry 39:1233–1241, 1982

Bridges-Parlet S, Knopman D, Thompson T: A descriptive study of physically aggressive behavior in dementia by direct observation. J Am Geriatr Soc 42:192–197, 1994

Brown GL, Goodwin FK, Ballenger JC, et al: Aggression in humans correlates with cerebrospinal fluid amine metabolites. Psychiatry Res 1:131–139, 1979

Bushman BJ, Cooper HM: Effects of alcohol on human aggression: an integrative research review. Psychol Bull 107:341–354, 1990

Cases O, Seif I, Grimsby J, et al: Aggressive behavior and altered amounts of brain serotonin and norepinephrine in mice lacking MAOA. Science 268(5218):1763–1766, 1995

Castellanos RX, Elia J, Kruesi MJ, et al: Cerebrospinal fluid monamine metabolites in boys with attention-deficit hyperactivity disorder. Psychiatry Res 52:305–316, 1994

Centers for Medicare and Medicaid Services: Seclusion and restraint for behavior management (§482.13[f]), in Hospital Conditions of Participation for Patients' Rights: Interpretive Guidelines. Baltimore, MD, Centers for Medicare and Medicaid Services, 1999

Chouinard G, Amable L, Turnier L, et al: A double-blind randomized clinical trial of rapid tranquilization with i.m. clonazepam and i.m. haloperidol in agitated psychotic patients with manic symptoms. Can J Psychiatry 38 (suppl 4):S114–S121, 1993

Christmas AJ, Maxwell DR: A comparison of the effects of some benzodiazepines and other drugs on aggressive and exploratory behaviour in mice and rats. Neuropharmacology 9:17–29, 1970

Citrome L, Volavka J: Violent patients in the emergency setting. Psychiatr Clin North Am 22:789–801, 1999

Coccaro EF: Central serotonin and impulsive aggression. Br J Psychiatry Suppl 8:52–62, 1989

Coccaro EF: Impulsive aggression and central serotonergic system function in humans: an example of a dimensional brain-behavioral relationship. Int Clin Psychopharmacol 7:3–12, 1992

Coccaro EF, Siever LJ, Klar HM, et al: Serotonergic studies in patients with affective and personality disorders. Arch Gen Psychiatry 46: 587–599, 1989

Cohen-Mansfield J, Billig N: Agitated behaviors in the elderly: a conceptual review. J Am Geriatr Soc 34:711–721, 1986

Convit A, Nemes ZC, Volavka J: History of phencyclidine use and repeated assaults in newly admitted young schizophrenic men (letter). Am J Psychiatry 145:1176, 1988

Crowner ML (ed): Understanding and Treating Violent Psychiatric Patients. Washington, DC, American Psychiatric Press, 2000

Currier GW: Atypical antipsychotic medications in the psychiatric emergency service. J Clin Psychiatry 61 (suppl 14): 21–26, 2000

Currier GW, Allen MH: American Association for Emergency Psychiatry survey, I: psychiatric emergency service structure and function. Presented at the 51st American Psychiatric Association Institute on Psychiatric Services, New Orleans, LA, October 29–November 2, 1999

Dabbs JM Jr, Carr TS, Frady RL, et al: Testosterone, crime, and misbehavior among 692 male prison inmates. Personality and Individual Differences 18:627–633, 1995

Donlon PT, Hopkin JT, Tupin JT, et al: Haloperidol for acute schizophrenic patients: an evaluation of three oral regimens. Arch Gen Psychiatry 37:691–695, 1980

Dorevitch A, Katz N, Zemishlany Z, et al: Intramuscular flunitrazepam versus intramuscular haloperidol in the emergency treatment of aggressive psychotic behavior. Am J Psychiatry 156:142–144, 1999

Eronen M, Angermeyer MC, Schulze B: The psychiatric epidemiology of violent behaviour. Soc Psychiatry Psychiatr Epidemiol 33(suppl): S13–S23, 1998

Estroff SE, Swanson JW, Lachicotte WS, et al: Risk reconsidered: targets of violence in the social networks of people with serious psychiatric disorders. Social Psychiatry Psychiatr Epidemiol 33 (suppl 1):S95–S101, 1998

Germine M., Goddard AW, Woods SW, et al: Anger and anxiety responses to m-CPP in GAD. Biol Psychiatry 32:457–461, 1992

Gerra G, Zaimovic A, Avanzini P, et al: Neurotransmitter-neuroendocrine responses to experimentally induced aggression in humans: influence of personality variable. Psychiatry Res 66:33–43, 1997

Gogos JA, Morgan M, Luine V, et al: Catechol-O-methyltransferase-deficient mice exhibit sexually dimorphic changes in catecholamine levels and behavior. Proc Natl Acad Sci U S A 95:9991–9996, 1998

Grafman J, Schwab K, Warden D, et al: Frontal lobe injuries, violence, and aggression: a report of the Vietnam Head Injury Study. Neurology 46:1231–1238, 1996

Hallikainen T, Saito T, Lachman HM, et al: Association between low activity serotonin transporter promoter genotype with habitual impulsive behavior among antisocial early onset alcoholics. Mol Psychiatry 4(4):385-388, 1999

Haug M, Simler S, Kim L, et al: Studies on the involvement of GABA in the aggression directed by groups of intact or gonadectomized male and female mice towards lactating intruders. Pharmacol Biochem Behav 12:189–193, 1980

Heinrichs RW: Frontal cerebral lesions and violent incidents in chronic neuropsychiatric patients. Biol Psychiatry 25:174–178, 1989

Hirschi T, Hindelang MJ: Intelligence and delinquency: a revisionist review. American Sociological Review 42:571–587, 1977

Hodgins S: Mental disorder, intellectual deficiency, and crime: evidence from a birth cohort. Arch Gen Psychiatry 49:476–483, 1992

Joint Commission on Accreditation of Healthcare Organizations: 2002 Hospital Accreditation Standards. Oakbrook Terrace, IL, Joint Commission Resources, 2002

Kahn MW: A comparison of personality, intelligence, and social history of two criminal groups. J Soc Psychol 49:33–40, 1959.

Klassen D, O'Connor W: A prospective study of predictors of violence in adult male mental patients. Law and Human Behavior 12:143–158, 1998

Lachman HM, Nolan KA, Mohr P, et al: Association between catechol O-methyltransferase genotype and violence in schizophrenia and schizoaffective disorder. Am J Psychiatry 155:835–837, 1998

Lamprecht F, Eichelman B, Thoa NB, et al: Rat fighting behavior: serum dopamine-β-hydroxylase and hypothalamic tyrosine hydroxylase. Science 177:1214–1215, 1972

Langevin R, Ben-Aron M, Wortzman G, et al: Brain damage, diagnosis, and substance abuse among violent offenders. Behav Sci Law 5:77–94, 1987

Lidz CW, Mulvey EP, Gardner W: The accuracy of predictions of violence to others. JAMA 269:1007–1011, 1993

Lindenmayer JP: The pathophysiology of agitation. J Clin Psychiatry 61 (suppl 14):5–10, 2000

Lindenmayer JP, Kotsaftis A: Use of sodium valproate in violent and aggressive behaviors: a critical review. J Clin Psychiatry 61(2):123–128, 2000

Linnoila M, Virkkunen M, Scheinin M, et al: Low cerebrospinal fluid 5-hydroxyindoleacetic acid concentration differentiates impulsive from nonimpulsive violent behavior. Life Sci 33:2609–2614, 1983

Mann JJ, Stanley M, McBride PA, et al: Increased serotonin$_2$ and β-adrenergic receptor binding in the frontal cortices of suicide victims. Arch Gen Psychiatry 43(10):954–959, 1986

McKinlay WW, Brooks DN, Bond MR, et al: The short-term outcome of severe blunt head injury as reported by relatives of the injured persons. J Neurol Neurosurg Psychiatry 44:527–533, 1981

Meehan K, Zhang F, David S, et al: A double-blind, randomized comparison of the efficacy and safety of intramuscular injections of olanzapine, lorazepam or placebo in threatening acutely agitated patients diagnosed with bipolar mania. J Clin Psychopharmacology 21: 389–397, 2001

Mintzer J, Brawman-Mintzer O, Mirski DF, et al: Fenfluramine challenge test as a marker of serotonin activity in patients with Alzheimer's dementia and agitation. Biol Psychiatry 44(9):918–921, 1998

Moffitt TE, Silva PA: Neuropsychological deficit and self-reported delinquency in an unselected birth cohort. J Am Acad Child Adolesc Psychiatry 27:233–240, 1988

Moller SE, Mortensen EL, Breun L, et al: Aggression and personality: association with amino acids and monoamine metabolites. Psychol Med 26:323–331, 1996

Monahan J, Steadman HJ, Silver E, et al: Rethinking Risk Assessment: The MacArthur Study of Mental Disorder and Violence. New York, Oxford University Press, 2001

Moyer KE: The Psychobiology of Aggression. New York, Harper & Row, 1976

New AS, Gelernter J, Yovell Y, et al: Tryptophan hydroxylase genotype is associated with impulsive-aggression measures. Am J Med Genet 81:13–17, 1998

Newhill CE, Mulvey EP, Lidz CW: Characteristics of violence in the community by female patients seen in a psychiatric emergency room. Psychiatr Serv 46:785–789, 1995

Nielsen DA, Goldman D, Virkkunen M, et al: Suicidality and 5-hydroxyindoleacetic acid concentration associated with a tryptophan hydroxylase polymorphism. Arch Gen Psychiatry 51:34–38, 1994

Nordt SP, Clark RF: Midazolam: a review of therapeutic uses and toxicity. J Emerg Med 15(3):357–365, 1997

Puglisi-Allegra S: Effects of sodium n-dipropylacetate, muscimol hydrobromide and (R,S) nipecotic acid amide on isolation-induced aggressive behavior. Psychopharmacology (Berl) 70:287–290, 1980

Raine A, Meloy JR, Bihrle S et al: Reduced prefrontal and increased subcortical brain functioning assessed using positron emission tomography in predatory and affective murderers. Behav Sci Law 16:319–332, 1998

Randall LO, Schallek W, Heise GA, et al: The psychosedative properties of methaminodiazepoxide. J Pharmacol Clin Ther 129:163–171, 1960

Ratey JJ, Sorgi P, O'Driscoll GA, et al: Nadolol to treat aggression and psychiatric symptomatology in chronic psychiatric inpatients: a double-blind, placebo-controlled study. J Clin Psychiatry 53:41–46, 1992

Sachdev P, Kruk J: Restlessness: the anatomy of a neuropsychiatric symptom. Aust N Z J Psychiatry 30:38–53, 1996

Salzman C, Solomon D, Miyawaki E, et al: Parenteral lorazepam versus parenteral haloperidol for the control of psychotic disruptive behavior. J Clin Psychiatry 52(4):177–180, 1991

Schatzberg A, DeBattista C: Phenomenology and treatment of agitation. J Clin Psychiatry 60 (suppl 15):17–20, 1999

Silver E, Mulver EP, Monahan J: Assessing violence risk among discharged psychiatric patients: toward an ecological approach. Law and Human Behavior 23:235–253, 1999

Simler S, Puglisi-Allegra S, Mandel P: Effects of n-dipropylacetate on aggressive behavior and brain GABA level in isolated mice. Pharmacol Biochem Behav 18:717–720, 1983

Soininen H, McDonald H, Rekonen M, et al: Homovanillic acid and 5-hydroxyindoleacetic acid levels in CSF in patients with senile dementia of Alzheimer type. Acta Neurol Scand 64:101–107, 1981

Spellacy F: Neuropsychological discrimination between violent and nonviolent men and adolescents. J Clin Psychol 34:49–52, 1978

Steadman HJ, Cocozza JJ, Melick ME: Explaining the increased arrest rate among mental patients: the changing clientele of state hospitals. Am J Psychiatry 135:816–820, 1978

Strous RD, Bark N, Parsia SS, et al: Analysis of a functional catechol O-methyltransferase gene polymorphism in schizophrenia: evidence for association with aggressive and antisocial behavior. Psychiatry Res 69:71–77, 1997

Stueve A, Link BG: Violence and psychiatric disorders: results from an epidemiological study of young adults in Israel. Psychiatr Q 68(4): 327–342, 1997

Swartz MS, Swanson JW, Hiday VA, et al: Violence and severe mental illness: the effects of substance abuse and nonadherence to medication. Am J Psychiatry 155(2):226–231, 1998

Tariot PN: Treatment of agitation and dementia. J Clin Psychiatry 60 (suppl 8):11–20, 1999

Taylor PJ: When symptoms of psychosis drive serious violence. Soc Psychiatry Psychiatr Epidemiol 33(suppl):S47–S54, 1998

Träskman-Bendz L, Alling C, Oreland L, et al: Prediction of suicidal behavior from biologic tests. J Clin Psychopharmacol 12:215–265, 1992

Valzelli L: Activity of benzodiazepines on aggressive behavior in rats and mice, in The Benzodiazepines. Edited by Garattini S, Mussini E, Randall LO. New York, Raven, 1973, pp 405–417

Virkkunen M: Insulin secretion during the glucose tolerance test among habitually violent and impulsive offenders. Aggress Behav 12:303–310, 1986

Virkkunen M, Nuutila A, Goodwin FK, et al: Cerebrospinal fluid monoamine metabolites in male arsonists. Arch Gen Psychiatry 44:241–247, 1987

Volavka J: Neurobiology of Violence. Washington, DC, American Psychiatric Press, 1995

Wessely S: The Camberwell Study of Crime and Schizophrenia. Soc Psychiatry Psychiatr Epidemiol 33(suppl):S24–S28, 1998

Williams D: Neural factors related to habitual aggression. Brain 95:503–520, 1969

Wong MTH, Lumsden J, Fenton GW, et al: Electroencephalography, computed tomography and violence ratings of male patients in a maximum-security mental hospital. Acta Psychiatr Scand 90:97–101, 1994

Wyant M, Diamond B, O'Neal E, et al: The use of midazolam in acutely agitated psychiatric patients. Psychopharmacol Bull 26:126–129, 1990

Yeudall LT: Neuropsychological assessment of forensic disorder. Canada's Mental Health 25:7–15, 1977

Chapter 5

Psychosocial Interventions in the Psychiatric Emergency Service

A Skills Approach

Ronald C. Rosenberg, M.D.
Kerry J. Sulkowicz, M.D.

In this chapter, we consider the acquisition of skills necessary to deal with psychosocial and psychotherapeutic issues in emergency mental health. Whereas the role of the psychiatric emergency service (PES) in providing gatekeeping functions, including assessment, diagnosis, stabilization, and disposition, is well established (Forster 1994; Gerson 1980), its role as a care setting—and, in particular, a psychotherapy setting—is more controversial. Historically, PESs have operated as triage services; the goal has been to provide only the assessment and care necessary to place the patient in another setting. It has been common to lament the PES environment as antitherapeutic (Gerson 1980; Langs 2000). However, as the scope of assessment and pharmacological treatment in emergency settings has grown (Allen 2001), others have begun to address the psychotherapeutic elements intrinsic to the PES's expanded mission (Berlin 2000; Kass and Karasu 1979; Rosenberg and Kesselman 1993; Thienhaus 1995).

Even triage requires that certain minimum procedures be completed in a timely manner, and certain interpersonal skills help to accomplish those procedures. However, some staff attitudes and behaviors can be inflammatory and detrimental to the process. More ambitiously, a crisis can be thought of as an opportunity for staff to engage the patient, for the patient to experience the episode as helpful, and, ideally, for some change to occur. Philosophically, this chapter is predicated on the assumption that crisis services can and should do more than simply gather the data necessary to send patients elsewhere. Both staff and patients benefit from this posture. This chapter is devoted to a discussion of the interpersonal processes that occur between patients and staff in emergencies and the ways in which these may be used to enhance the professional's understanding of the patient and the patient's sense of benefit from the encounter. Another assumption is that patients will often have many encounters over a lifetime. Viewed in this way, a given encounter need not yield immediate results but should at least deliver a consistent message about the nature of mental health problems and the way they are approached.

Goals of Psychosocial Intervention in Emergencies

The first goal in emergencies is *safety,* and interpersonal awareness and skills are clearly related to safely engaging patients who are in crisis. The second goal is *assessment.* Observation of the patient's mode of relating to others and the reactions of others to the patient can be informative. This level of understanding is required for a more thorough formulation of the patient's difficulties and is necessary to realistically assist the patient in dealing with the external world. Finally, in some cases, it may be possible to facilitate slight but meaningful *changes in the patient's internal world.*

Linear Procedure Versus Flexible Process

The work of the PES can be understood in terms of discrete procedures that must ultimately be completed by staff for all encounters versus processes that appear to occur spontaneously. In general, the procedures entail interviews that operationalize lists of symptoms, risk factors, and so forth. At one extreme, the interviewer may emphasize compliance with linear completion of the symptom checklist and offer an opinion as to where the patient should go for help with the problems described. Emotional reactions of patients in this case may be viewed as evidence of illness or ignored as noncontributory. This will be referred to as the *procedural approach*, because it is dominated by attention to the procedure, not the patient. Linear adherence to procedures may be associated with high procedural fidelity but poor outcome because it is devoted not to the needs of the patient but to the needs of the staff.

Alternatively, assessments usually begin with open-ended inquiries about the reason for the presentation, at which point clinicians begin to apply more or less structure, depending on the patient's needs and characteristics and the current state of the PES environment (e.g., time pressure, privacy). Clinicians in this situation exhibit flexibility about departures from the checklist. They attend to the emotional reactions of the patient to the topics under discussion and to the manner in which the patient relates to the examiner. Through awareness of these elements of the process of the interview, they begin to develop theories about the patient that they then test in some way that is not necessarily related to the explicit focus of the interview at all.

Such a *process approach* may include a variety of psychotherapeutic interventions, in which the selection of technique is guided partly by the nature of the patient's presentation and partly by the orientation, training, and experience of the staff member. The same questions may ultimately be answered, but the more tools and time available to the clinician, the more likely the patient will feel that the conversation has met his or her needs. The more complex process approach may then ultimately decrease the patient's frustration and aggressivity and improve compliance with the required procedures. It may also contribute to motivating patients to pursue or continue treatment after discharge.

It should be noted that the milieu of most emergency services is focused on efficiency and control in a way that may not seem to support a process approach to patients. Time, space, and privacy are limited. The physical arrangement of beds, chairs, rooms, and so forth is usually quite different from that of a clinic or a private office. Care is often initiated in an atmosphere of crisis and coercion, resulting in pressures not found in other settings. Consequently, it is necessary to *modify* therapeutic principles developed in more ordered milieus in order to adapt them to the pressures of the PES.

Psychosocial Interventions in Psychiatric Emergencies

It can be said that there are three phases or components of psychosocial intervention that may occur in emergency settings. The first is *building an alliance*. The second is *dealing with the crisis driving the presentation through some form of stabilization or intervention*. The third is *introducing elements of psychotherapy*.

Therapeutic Alliance

The therapeutic alliance refers to the psychoanalytic concept (Bibring 1937; Zetzel 1956) of the belief by the patient, both conscious and unconscious, that the work of therapy will benefit him or her. There is a tacit acknowledgment that something is wrong and an implicit willingness or capability of enduring some discomfort during treatment, often, but not limited to, an increase in anxiety. Poor alliances predict poorer outcomes (Clarkin et al. 1987). Poor alliances also predict greater violence after the patient is admitted (Beauford et al. 1997).

Factors in Establishing the Therapeutic Alliance

How does one improve the likelihood of getting the cooperation of patients to endure the lists of questions intrinsic to the work of the PES? When can crisis work begin? When will the patient accept healing and direction? Literature has been accumulating on the central role of the therapeutic alliance in psychotherapy (Luborsky et al. 1983; Marziali et al. 1981). Often, establishing an alliance precedes or facilitates needed crisis intervention and the acceptance of healing and direction.

The lead author's research (Rosenberg 1995; Rosenberg and

Kesselman 1993) indicates that there are factors increasing the likelihood that alliances can be built and, equally important, that there are even more factors destructive of the alliance building that need to be overcome. Of particular interest is the presence of psychotic features, which tend to decrease alliance potential until these symptoms are controlled (Kane et al. 1983). Also, being brought by family members, by police, or by ambulance has negative consequences. It is not unusual for all three features to be present. If one is self-referred, the chances for success improve dramatically. Surprisingly, the presence of substance abuse frequently has positive implications regarding the alliance.

Building an Alliance

Alliance building is critical regardless of the modality of treatment that is indicated. This work is usually recommended or required in the first phase of the emergency room contact; however, with agitated patients, it is sometimes accomplished after the patient is calmer. Although implicit from the initial contact with the patient, the alliance-building work proceeds throughout the interview. Although some staff intuitively build therapeutic alliances, several specific techniques can be helpful:

1. *Attend to the patient's concrete needs.* If the patient is hungry, thirsty, or sleepy, attempt to meet these needs or allow the patient a sense of token gratification by at least acknowledging these needs.
2. *Use* alliance-building *questions in the early phase of the assessment and postpone potentially* alliance-deflecting *questions to later in the interview.*
3. *In general, use questions that promote the alliance.* Such questions are directed at helping patients identify and describe their distressing experiences without compromising their sense of self-efficacy and self-esteem. Neutral questions presented in a supportive manner work best.

    Depending on the circumstances, alliance-building questions might include

    - Have you been sleeping well?
    - Are you in any physical discomfort?

- How has your appetite been lately? Has your weight changed?
- Have you been feeling sad or upset lately? Tell me about what has been upsetting you.
- What do you do to make yourself feel good? Movies? TV? Friends? Sports? Have you found that you are less interested in these activities lately?
- Have other people been upsetting you? Could you explain some of this to me?

Ultimately, questions, such as those below, must be posed that may reveal embarrassing deficits, that reflect negatively on the patient in some way, or that may seem trivial in the face of the patient's distress. In some cases, these questions may be at the center of the presentation and may need to be addressed early; however, if possible, these may be postponed or at least put into context.

- What is today's date?
- Are you hearing voices?
- Did you ever use cocaine?
- Can you subtract 7 from 100?
- Have you had legal difficulties?

4. *Demonstrate empathy.* Make supportive statements even in the face of provocation: "This has been a difficult day for you." "I can understand how this is hard for you." Note how the patient reacts to these statements. Despite occasional angry responses, there is often an unconscious softening response, in which the patient begins to see the staff as potentially helpful.

5. *Help debrief some of the emotionally toxic aspects of the emergency room referral or even previous therapy* (Kass and Karasu 1979; Meyerson et al. 1998; Rabkin 1977). If the patient was brought by force or required restraint or intramuscular medication, it can be helpful to acknowledge how unpleasant that experience can be: "It must have been frightening when the police brought you here." "I know you didn't want to come here, but perhaps we can help you if I could ask a few questions."

6. *Directly or indirectly inquire about feelings about therapy and illness.* The following questions are useful:

- Do you think that you have an illness or emotional problem with which you need help?
- What do you think is the problem?
- Do you think medications might help?
- Would it help to talk to a professional in confidence about things that are troubling you?
- Would being in the hospital [if this seems likely] help you with your problems?

The alliance-building process will proceed regardless of the immediate responses of patient. The examiner should make note of but not be distressed by the gap between the patient's representation of the problems and objective reality. In fact, all the information provided by the patient at this stage may be obviously false.

Note that irritability and a brusque or condescending manner in the examiner have the potential to traumatize or retraumatize the patient and can undermine alliance-building efforts, leading to mutual frustration and therapeutic stalemate. There is evidence that an irritable style can increase assault potential for the interviewer and other staff members (Black et al. 1994). Awareness of one's own affective state—for example, fatigue from a night on call, anxiety about a personal matter, or anger and frustration regarding training—is critical when one is approaching PES patients. A moment of self-calming, even a deep breath, can have a beneficial impact on one's interaction with patients.

Observing or reflecting on the effect of their own body language and voice tone on the process can help staff in stressful situations, such as when they are talking down an agitated patient or encouraging a mute patient to respond.

Crisis Intervention: A Dual Approach

Another universal feature of psychosocial interventions in the PES is the presence of acute or recent stressors prior to the PES visit. Although many of these may be related to exacerbation of long-standing emotional problems, dealing with these issues is necessary and, for some, the essence of the PES service.

This crisis approach has been defined by Caplan (1964). A crisis is provoked when a person faces an obstacle (hazard) to important life goals that is for the time insurmountable through the utilization of customary methods of problem solving behavior (coping behavior). During the ensuing period of disorganization (the crisis) a variety of abortive attempts are made to solve the problem. Eventually some kind of adaptation is achieved which may or may not be in the best interest of that person or his fellows.

The crisis model assumes that the patient was previously in a state of *equilibrium* and analyzes what is needed to *restore* equilibrium.

The crisis formulation is nonmedical, and this type of assessment and intervention operates in parallel with medical-model diagnosis and treatment. Depression, psychotic thinking, and chronic personality traits may interfere with crisis intervention and render it ineffective and even counterproductive. Thus, typical PES work involves two phases—sometimes simultaneous, sometimes parallel, and sometimes cyclical: 1) stabilization of the patient and 2) identification and resolution or partial resolution of the crisis.

This process may involve simply replacing or reinforcing internal or external assets and returning to the previous equilibrium or status quo. This limited compensatory effort might be referred to as stabilization. On the other hand, dealing with the crisis may involve the acquisition of new understanding or new cognitive or interpersonal skills or the modification of relationships by which a new and potentially better equilibrium is reached. To the extent that the goal is for the patient to change in some way, the effort moves beyond stabilization to therapy.

Therapy Work

The previous two sections dealt with two processes found in virtually all PES psychosocial interventions: building an alliance and assessing and implementing crisis intervention involving material and tangible assistance. We now turn to a critical third component, *therapy work*. The bulk of this work involves exchanging thoughts and language (including sign language and body language statements) between the patient and the staff so that the patient is better able to negotiate the crisis and resume functioning. This work can draw on a diverse number of potential schools of therapy, sometimes with conflicting objectives, such as behavioral, cognitive, cognitive-behavioral, dynamic, and family systems approaches and, more recently, psychoeducational efforts. The goal of alliance building is to *engage,* and the goal of crisis stabilization is to *assist.* In both of these approaches it is assumed that the patient will simply return to a previous level of functioning. The goal of therapy is to produce enduring *change,* even if only by increments.

The goals of therapeutic change in the PES are generally modest but may be meaningful in a larger context for the patient. The overall goal should be reducing the likelihood that the crisis necessitating an emergency room visit or admission will recur. Such objectives for the patient include changing current thinking, introducing new thinking, and acquiring new knowledge about the self or emotional illness or, in some cases, about substance abuse. Other objectives include examining impulse, linking thoughts to appropriate actions or inhibiting inappropriate actions, and learning how to make better decisions. Sometimes an objective is simply learning how to label affects or to recognize unusual or disturbed thoughts. Interpersonal objectives can include learning to communicate with others more appropriately, learning how to assert oneself, and learning to listen to the communication of others more accurately.

One challenge in PES therapy work is that many characteristics of therapies in the office setting do not apply to the PES. In fact, an examination of the criteria for a variety of short-term therapies lists exclusionary criteria that would eliminate 95% of a typical PES population (Crits-Christoph and Barber 1991). The milieu of the PES is noisy, with minimal privacy and overlapping staff roles that can be confusing to the patient. Referrals to the PES typically have a coercive component, and treatment is severely compressed. In some places, patients are expected to be seen and issues are expected to be resolved within hours; in others, 2 or 3 days are permitted at most. There is little time for the building of therapeutic relationships; nor is there always consistency of approach among staff.

Nevertheless, regardless of staff's personal, professional, or institutional theoretical orientation, some aspect of virtually every therapeutic approach can be useful in the PES, particularly if the clinician remains flexible and has modest goals. Thus, a large number of staff, even with contradictory theories and goals, can be helpful in a PES setting.

Although a trial of therapy is instructive, monitoring anxiety tolerance is critical (Davanloo 1979). There is a key rule akin to the notion of "Safety first": Always observe the patient for anxiety, agitation, and psychosis as you proceed and be prepared to modify or abandon your technique, *including stopping the interview* if your patient shows signs of going over a reasonable threshold, which is usually lower than that acceptable in an office setting.

There is no substitute for experience in understanding where that threshold is. Many therapy techniques uncover hidden psychological material. This sometimes results in immediate or delayed agitation. The patient's capacity to tolerate anxiety and curb impulsivity is initially unknown and may have been modified by concurrent illness, drug abuse, acute or chronic psychosis, the emergence of a mood episode, insomnia, hunger, pain, metabolic instability, or acute psychological or physical trauma. Speaking to others who know the patient, consulting with other staff members, and considering manifest behavior in the PES are always indicated before proceeding with a therapeutic intervention. Furthermore, because of subtle differences in dress, manner, intonation, body stance, (possibly) age, interpersonal distance, physical use of space, language, and perceived power, the very same tactic that succeeds for one person may fail with another. Finally, irritability, impatience, and careless language will have untoward effects, as mentioned in the subsection on alliance building.

In general, there are three schools of therapy work applicable in the PES: behavioral, cognitive, and dynamic. Psychoeducational, family, and cultural approaches are also important, but these may be viewed as modifiers of the first triad. Combining approaches should be viewed as desirable, rather than as a compromise, and often renders the treatment more robust and flexible. The majority of patients will have received medication, which can increase the efficiency and safety of psychotherapeutic interventions, provided patients are not too sedated or distracted by unpleasant side effects. Although the milieu and medication frequently can set the initial agenda, the persistent therapist can usually engage the patient in dealing with other substantive issues.

In what follows, we review, for illustrative purposes, examples of common schools of treatment and give some indication of useful modifications and limitations.

Behavioral Approaches

Behavior therapy principles as advocated by Wolpe and Lazarus (Wolpe 1990) are usually valuable to consider, but classic office techniques of flooding and abreaction, which raise anxiety levels (see Wolpe 1990, Chapter 10), should be avoided. When patients are agitated, hostile, and unable to exchange thoughts and language, a behavioral approach is particularly useful, especially when coupled with medications. Such an approach may be a potent positive reinforcer that motivates patients to improve.

> **Patient:** Get me out of here!! I'll get you!
> **Staff:** Please calm down sir. Perhaps we can help you.
> **Patient:** You can't help me! You just want to make money!
> **Staff:** Perhaps we should talk later when you are feeling better. *(Staff backs away.)*
> **Patient:** No come back, I want to talk to you. I want out!
> **Staff:** Can you tell us a little about—
> **Patient** *(interrupting):* Just get me out of here! Don't ask me questions! I'm not answering questions!
> **Staff** *(moving away again):* If you can remain calm for a few moments, I will return. *(Patient becomes a bit quieter.)*

Sometimes this dialogue repeats several times. Not uncommonly, medication is administered in this cycle; yet certain unscripted behavioral therapeutic paradigms play an important role in rewarding the patient for self-control. To maximize the sense of reward, however, the staff should not appear angry or apprehensive. Other reinforcers, such as access to other patients, cigarettes (in some facilities), and television, can be used in a systematic way to influence behavior.

Beyond acute management, using desensitization, with the cycle of evoking distressing thoughts and then making calming statements, and encouraging patients to use relaxation techniques are what Wolpe (1990) calls "Counter-Anxiety Responses" and can be valuable.

A 56-year-old self-referred man with schizophrenia taking clozapine presented with increased agitation and paranoia, describing how he was assaulted near a public bus:

> **Patient:** I got up from my seat and paid my fare and this guy follows me . . . *(pauses and shakes restlessly)*
> **Staff** *(interrupting):* This is upsetting you. Can you take a breath. *(Patient, imitating the therapist, takes a breath.)*
> **Patient:** I was really scared. I knew something bad was going to happen. He says "You took my money! . . ."
> **Staff** *(interrupting as patient becomes more agitated):* Okay, okay. Hold it. Try this. Try to sit in the chair and just let your arms hang down. *(Patient complies.)* Are you ready to continue?
> **Patient:** Yeah . . . So I say, "No I didn't!"

Cognitive Approaches

Cognitive approaches (Beck and Greenberg 1979) involve a directness that is useful in PES work; such approaches are most suitable for patients with relatively intact cognitive functioning. Hence, a cognitive screen should be done before variants of these techniques are used (Copersino et al. 1998). Although psychosis does not absolutely preclude their use, understanding the meaning of a patient's communications and ensuring that a patient understands the therapist's response are important. Psychotic patients who are experiencing a crisis, once they have been stabilized with medication, can gain from this approach. Again, the "Goldilock's Rule" of not too much anxiety, just the right amount, should be observed.

Albert Ellis's paradigm (Ellis 1973) of an *event* producing *beliefs* that foster *emotional consequences* suggests the therapeutic strategy of attempting to *disrupt* the old belief to effect new feelings. Ellis's disruption involves the use of challenge, and challenge begets anxiety and sometimes hostility and irritability. Beck (1976) uses a more Socratic method that can be more palatable to patients and staff. He looks for evidence of *automatic thinking*, an important concept we will consider with the work of Donald Meichenbaum later in this section. Beck considers patient beliefs "biased" rather than "irrational," and therefore there is an attempt to mediate between what the therapist believes and what the patient believes. Consider the "seven deadly sins" of negative automatic thinking and some typical PES interventions.

1. Catastrophizing:

   Patient: My business is ruined. My marriage is ruined. My life is over. [inappropriate conclusion]

2. Selective abstraction:

   Patient: I went to the dance and no one would talk to me. I am a social failure. [unwarranted generalization]

3. Overgeneralization:

   Patient: Men are awful. No one can be trusted.

4. Magnification:

   Patient: This is the worst thing that can happen to me!

5. Personalization:

   Patient: I am totally to blame for this!

6. Labeling and mislabeling:

   Patient: I am a failure. I can't do anything right!

7. Polarized thinking:

   Patient: There is nothing good about this at all.

Staff should be alert to words and phrases like "all," "very," "the worst," and "my fault." Correcting these cognitive distortions takes careful and attentive listening and patience. Staff should not feel compelled to complete the job, as it is sufficient to begin helping the patient to think differently. Labeling maladaptive thinking per se is useful and can be done soon after an initial assessment. Observe how patients respond to this. Not infrequently, the patient is amused, confused, or only mildly irritated but not hostile or challenging. In fact, patients who become agitated when gentle support is offered are manifesting important diagnostic signs that can be hidden during a traditional structured interview.

Examples of gentle challenge to dysfunctional thinking applicable to the PES are as follows:

- "I hear what you say, but I find this kind of thinking upsetting. Is there another way to think about this?"
- "It has to be hard to live with all these negative thoughts."
- "How long have you thought this way? Was there a time when you thought differently?"

Before leaving the arena of cognitive-behavioral treatments, mention needs to be made of Meichenbaum's concept of cognitive-behavioral modification (CBM) (Meichenbaum 1972, 1977). Meichenbaum looked at the internal maladaptive speech of hyperactive children. For example, whereas a child who is frustrated might be having a thought like "I can't wait until class ends," a child with an attention deficit might have no thought at all and simply be making growling sounds or nonspecific noise. Thinking is conceptualized as a behavioral intermediary between stimulus and response that needs direction and/or correction. Further, maladaptive thoughts about the self yield maladaptive behaviors. Individuals with personality disorders often show evidence of this. Working not only to challenge dysfunctional thinking, as in the examples of Beck's work above, but to teach better thinking can be very helpful, assuming that the patient can begin to internalize these thoughts. Again, cognitive capacity is important.

> **Patient:** I want to leave now. I am a prisoner here.
> **Staff:** How can I know it is safe for you to go? You told us that you wanted to kill yourself. That you are no good. Tell me what has changed.

Patient: I just want to go back to work.

Staff: That's good. What will you do when you get back to work.

Patient: Nothing. Just go back to work.

Staff: Will you tell your supervisor about that incident that upset you? You seem to think you deserve . . .

Patient: Yes. I should ask for . . .

Staff: Okay. How would you do that?

Again, watch carefully for signs of anxiety, psychotic distortions, and agitation as a new script is created to replace a dysfunctional one.

Dynamic Approaches

Psychodynamic interventions add additional layers to assessment, encompassing a historical perspective that can inform diagnosis. Understanding long-enduring patterns of relatedness, chronic maladaptive traits, and recalled historical data may provide useful clues to evolving patterns of illness as opposed to the onset of new symptoms.

Dynamic psychiatry, which owes its legacy to Sigmund Freud (Bergman and Hartman 1976) and his followers, is based on the assumption that there are unconscious motivations that are screened from conscious awareness by defensive operations. Free association, transference/countertransference paradigms, and dream interpretation are some of the tools used by dynamically oriented therapists to explore the inner world of their patients.

A useful guide regarding dynamic interventions is to consider the exploratory-supportive intervention continuum (American Psychiatric Association 2001; Gabbard 2000). Supportive interventions can be incorporated into procedural approaches. These encompass affirmation, advice and praise, and empathic validation. As staff members acquire experience in process-related approaches, they can employ techniques of clarification, confrontation, or interpretation to help patients feel more comfortable with elaborating their histories. Formal definitions and some brief examples are cited below.

Supportive

Affirmation: Supporting the patient's comments and behavior.

Patient: I think I need to see someone to help me with my depression.
Therapist: That sounds like a good idea.

Advice and praise: Prescribing and reinforcing certain activities of benefit to the patient.

Patient: I am not going to use marijuana anymore.
Therapist: That's very good. Don't you think it would help to get treatment of your drug dependency?

Empathic validation: Demonstrating empathy with the patient's internal state.

Patient: I am feeling very depressed.
Therapist: It's understandable that the loss of your husband would make you feel that way.

Exploratory

Encouragement to elaborate: Requesting more information from the patient.

Patient: I am very angry at my mother.
Therapist: Can you tell me what she has done to upset you?

Clarification: Reformulating what the patient says into a more coherent view of what is relevant.

Patient: First he hits me, curses at me, and then steals my money. That's why I want to kill myself.
Therapist: It sounds like you feel humiliated and want to disappear.

Confrontation: Addressing issues the patient does not want to accept or wishes to avoid.

Patient: I just need a place to stay.
Therapist: Is it possible that you get thrown out by your parents because of your cocaine use? I wonder why you don't see that as a problem?

Interpretation: Linking a patient's feeling, thought, behavior, or symptom to its unconscious meaning or origin.

> **Patient:** If you don't admit me, I will kill myself.
> **Therapist:** Have you felt this way before?
> **Patient:** Sure, I've been suicidal before.
> **Therapist:** When was the last time? Does your regular therapist usually help with that?
> **Patient:** Yes, but I can't see her.
> **Therapist:** You describe her as very caring and wonderful but she's away. I wonder if you don't feel like an abandoned child who is angry at his mother for going away and would like us to care for you. What do you think?

As one progresses from supportive to exploratory interventions, greater clinician experience and attention to anxiety tolerance, as well as greater patient cognitive capacity and impulse control, are required. Nonetheless, certain patients in the PES will benefit most from the use of exploratory techniques in conjunction with crisis intervention.

While classic psychodynamic therapy may involve extended periods of time for the patient to develop stable and analyzable emotional reactions to the therapist (the transference), short-term versions began to emerge in the mid- to late 1970s (Marmor 1979). Sifneos (1979) used highly confrontational and anxiety-provoking questions to keep tensions high in a population of highly functional individuals who have little resemblance to the population that typically arrives at the PES. Others, such as Mann and Goldman (1982) and Malan (1976), developed short-term techniques that might serve a more diverse population.

Special populations, such as patients with borderline personality disorder, have particular problems that may result in PES visits. Intense affects, generated either by ongoing therapy or by patients' separation from their therapists, need to be understood in the context of an "emergency" (Adler 2000; Kass and Karasu 1979).

Mann and Goldman (1982) discussed the need to define a central focus for brief psychoanalytic work. Often this defined area of conflict is not what the patient had in mind when seeking therapy. It is here that the PES requires a departure from therapist-defined goals. The defined goals of any therapeutic intervention are dictated by *the circumstances that necessitated the visit in the first place.* Is the patient here because his therapist is away (abandonment issues)? Is the patient here because she is trying to get the therapist's attention (dependency issues)? Is the patient here because he lost his job and wants to commit suicide (competition; oedipal issues)? The dynamic work in the PES must reflect why the patient came. A common and important set of questions to ask the patient is "Why did you come for help now, as opposed to some other time?" "What is the emergency?" These simple questions are not simply the chief complaint but the entry point for most dynamic PES work.

Davanloo (1980), who introduced Intensive Short-term Dynamic Psychotherapy, developed more precise approaches to the situations described above that have broader applications. Among the concepts applicable in the PES are the "triangle of the person" and the "triangle of action." The person triangle involves mention of current persons in the patient's life, past persons in the patient's life, and the therapist (staff). The triangle of action describes the flux from anxiety to impulse to defense attached to one or more in the person triangle.

Patients can be asked the following questions during the early assessment:

From the triangle of the person:

- Where are your parents? (person of the distant past)
- Who raised you?
- Did you have friends when you were a child?

Then from the triangle of action:

- Did you get along with them? What were they like?
- How do you feel when you think of them?

Statements like "I hate (impulse-action triangle) my boss (current person-person triangle)" may be followed by anxiety or defensive operations. Understanding the types and levels of repetitive and maladaptive defenses is important in guiding future treatment, as well as in managing the patient in the PES. Higher-level defenses include intellectualization, sarcasm, reaction formation, and isolation of affect. Regressive defenses include defiance, denial, acting out, weepiness, passivity, aggression, projection, and dissociation.

As impulses are contained and defenses are challenged, other affects (and/or impulses) are released. This may enable further understanding and provide more appropriate targets for intervention.

There are other, less probing dynamic approaches to managing the PES patient. Lester Luborsky (1993) and others have written about the use of the therapist as an ally. Developing the concept of Short-Term Supportive Expressive Psychoanalytic Psychotherapy (Luborsky and David 1991), Luborsky builds on the therapeutic alliance, discussed earlier in this chapter, and attempts to frame symptoms as a way of coping. He is sensitive to the patient's need to test relationships and avoids long-winded and complex explanations.

In the PES, learning to trust and to relate to staff is an important therapeutic task. In the following example, the interviewer allies with the patient indirectly by engaging him in an exchange about the patient's reluctance to talk and his positive transference to another staff member.

> **Patient:** I don't want to talk about it.
> **Staff:** Is there anyone you've met here who you feel comfortable discussing this with?
> **Patient:** I liked the nurse who spoke to me when I came in.
> **Staff:** What did you like about her?
> **Patient:** She is like my aunt. I don't know.
> **Staff:** So you sort of trust her.
> **Patient:** Yeah, she's OK.

In outpatient therapy, anger might be seething but silent, whereas in the PES it might often be overt and could be displaced onto the PES visit itself. With such a patient, the following exchange might take place:

> **Patient:** I should not have come here. Everything takes too long.

Staff: We'll try to speed things up, but you can help by telling us a little about why you came.

Patient: I didn't want to come. It's my father's fault.

Staff: Can you tell us what happened.

Patient: No. That will take too long.

Staff: I wonder if you don't want to tell us because you are still angry with your father.

The patient's response at this point will likely reveal important clinical information about the patient's defensive style. Some possibilities are

Patient: Yes, you and him work together. [paranoia, projection]

Patient: Yes, he is nuts. He should be the one here. [splitting: good patient and staff, bad father]

Patient: I don't need to talk with you because I am really alright. [denial]

There are, of course, many other possible responses. If the patient is not too agitated, useful processing can take place and the staff gets a better understanding of the patient's style and capacity to adapt to the crisis. The father might be in the waiting area and might need to be directly engaged, not only for information about past treatments but as part of treatment in the family process. This leads us to consider, in the next section, the use of psychotherapy components in dealing with special situations such as family and interpersonal crises and the consequences of trauma.

Therapy Work for Special Situations

The Person and Person-Centered Therapy

Although difficult to classify, *person-centered therapy* offers an alternative way of conceiving styles of thinking. It involves taking an existential view of the patient as a person trying to live life, with all the events and forces that are often beyond the control of the individual. The emphasis is on "personhood" rather than "patienthood," that is, a nonmedical model in which patients are really clients and power is more equal. The central figure in this movement was Carl Rogers, whose seminal work *Client-Centered Therapy* (Rogers 1951; see also Rogers 1961) was a challenge to both behavioral and analytic approaches. "Rogerian" approaches can be approximated by a certain style of interviewing that involves intense empathic listening and repeating of what was heard.

> **Patient:** I didn't want to come here.
> **Therapist:** Yes, you didn't want to come here, but here you are.
> **Patient:** I had to do something.
> **Therapist:** It seems you made a decision to come here.

Richard Rabkin talks about how patients are demoralized, unsure of what is the matter, and have attempted strategies that have failed, yet they are unprepared for long-term treatment (Rabkin 1977, Chapter 1). A key component of this, as detailed by Talmon, is *empowerment*—that is, helping patients (clients) marshal forces within themselves that allow them to feel that they can solve their problems on their own. Talmon (1990, p.75) suggests questions such as

- What would you like to accomplish today?
- What will you do/feel/think when you don't need to come here anymore?
- How would you know when you have resolved this problem?

At the core of many decisions in the PES is an issue of responsibility—that is, someone must assume effective responsibility for ensuring at least a certain minimal outcome. Preferably the patient or a natural ally of the patient would be responsible throughout the episode. If not, then clinicians have the statutory authority to assume control in some circumstances. As a result, the power relationship is by definition unbalanced. Patients must wait to be seen and are told what to do. If necessary, they may be held and medicated against their will for their safety and the safety of others. Clarifying this issue and attempting to shift control to the patient under a defined set of circumstances can have a beneficial effect.

> **Patient:** I want to leave. I changed my mind. I really don't want to hurt anyone. I was just trying to get my girlfriend to listen to me. You can't keep me here against my will.

Therapist: You are right. If you were not really dangerous, I would have let you go. I can only keep you if you shout and show us how dangerous you are. If you can restrain yourself and talk to your girlfriend in a calm manner, I may be able to release you!

Notice how the power relationship is reframed such that the patient has power. A positive response may encourage further use of this paradigm. A negative reaction, on the other hand, may generate data that are valuable for understanding underlying illness.

Families and Networks

The emergence of family and network therapy has opened new opportunities for effective intervention in the PES. There are many models of family work (and network work). The PES visit can be an attempt by the individual to differentiate himself or herself, as described by the work of Murray Bowen (1978). It can be an opportunity for strategic change, as described in the work of Jay Haley (1977). It can lead to a greater sense of self-worth, in the mode of Virginia Satir (1983).

The alliance is more complex with families. Successful alliance building is predictive of success in office settings (Marziali et al. 1981), but in the PES it can prove problematic as people take sides. Patients often feel coerced to come to the PES and tend to have more initial negative views (Rosenberg and Kesselman 1993). No technique is effective in all circumstances, but a few are frequently helpful in building alliances with groups.

- *Determine who the leader is.* In a family network situation, the treating staff should try to assess who is dominant in the group. Sometimes building an alliance with the leader gives permission to the patient to continue treatment. This is generally the case with children. If the family leader is against treatment ("I don't want my son to have any medication!"), educating about, explaining, or reframing the treatment can result in less patient resistance to treatment and better cooperation.
- *Learn and deal with extreme views.* Deal openly and fairly with skepticism about treatment. On the other hand, moderate overly

idealistic and unreasonable expectations. Usually the most pessimistic person in the group will get attention. It is also possible that one member of the group will try to quietly sabotage treatment by saying little but sulking passively. It is vital to make sure everyone has a chance to contribute.

- *Be respectful of cultural issues.* Some cultures discourage introspection. Some only value somatic symptoms and treatments. There is a real element of negotiation involved in family and group work. Spiritual values should not be neglected.
- *Respect and advocate for your patient.* Under the stress of events leading to a PES visit, families and groups are less defended. Showing concern for the patient's physical and mental well-being is always alliance enhancing. Many of the same questions that are alliance building described earlier will also work in a group context (e.g., "Has your husband been sleeping well?" "When was the last time he had a physical examination?").
- *Watch and improve communication styles.* A number of family therapy schools emphasize communication styles (Whitaker and Malone 1981). Who speaks? Who is silent? Who says what? What is actually heard?

The family is an important resource for managing crises, but they also may contribute to the crisis. Hence, it may be essential to involve the family in order to resolve the crisis.

Giving useful information about resources, agencies, and prospective treatments to all members of the patient's network implicitly helps clarify roles and tends to decrease stress.

Observing the style of therapy work sometimes decreases suspicion and distortion of psychotherapy by some family members and facilitates continued care. Family groups provide an excellent opportunity to explain how treatments work (Van Gent and Zwart 1991; Wallace 1992). The following example demonstrates the alliance-building benefits of psychoeducational work with family members:

> **Father:** I don't want my son to be a zombie!
> **Staff:** Medication X does not cause that. However medication Y, which he will take at night, will help him sleep better so that he can do better the next day.

Father: I want him to keep his mind on his work.

Staff: Talking to the therapist could help him concentrate better, because he might be less distracted by thoughts that bother him.

Father: Well, you are the doctor.

Staff: Yes, and you are his father and he wants to please you. Could you help him to do these things?

Treatment of Trauma

Trauma is defined in terms of experiencing or witnessing threatening events with intense fear and helplessness. The diagnosis of posttraumatic disorder (PTSD) is highly specific, requiring trauma, persistent reexperiencing, avoidance of associated stimuli, and increased arousal. However, from a psychotherapeutic view, a more inclusive approach to trauma is useful. Not surprisingly, the PTSD patient can present to the PES long after occurrence of the trauma, often as a consequence of the disruptive effect of avoidance, impaired sleep, or use of drugs and alcohol as a way of coping. PTSD is often unrecognized at the time of a PES presentation unless there is specific inquiry made about traumatic experiences. It is also useful to observe for subtle signs of dissociation during the interviews and to enquire about milder forms of perceptual disturbance, such as derealization and depersonalization, rather than simply focusing exclusively on hallucinations.

Emphasis is now being placed on prevention in vulnerable individuals (Melancon and Boyer 1999). At the same time, the value of having patients debrief, retell, and relive their traumatic experience is being challenged (Wessely et al. 2000). While the issues are debated, PES patients will continue to arrive, some with an urgent need to talk about recent or past trauma, and others who are more reluctant or fearful to speak. The following suggestions are offered as an aid in working with trauma patients:

- *Take time to understand how the patient functioned prior to the traumatic event.* Enlist the help of collaterals to verify this. Assess to what extent avoidance behavior is in evidence.
- *Screen for and address any medical events or issues that could complicate coping.* These include brain injury, substance abuse,

endocrinopathy, complications of pregnancy or delivery, serious infections, and physical trauma or assault.

- *Assess the patient's general coping strategies.* The conceptualization of trauma as information overload (Horowitz 1991) would require responding to the patient's style of thinking. Kirtland et al. (1991) detailed how the approach to the patient varies with the patient's coping style (see below).
- *Be sensitive to the possible retraumatizing effect of the circumstances of the PES visit itself* (Meyerson 1998). Offer verbal support and an optimistic approach. On the other hand, no useful psychotherapy can be done with a panicky, agitated patient; hence, the use of medications and the use of strategies to decrease agitation and anxiety are valuable to the traumatized patient.

A history of trauma may put particular stress on the process of forming an alliance. Some traumas, including sexual assault, may be better handled with the involvement of a same-sex staff member. On occasion, a patient may express a preference for a therapist of the opposite sex, and this request should be honored if possible. Family and friends often are important intermediaries, facilitating trust. This can be especially true with paranoid patients, children, and some geriatric and adolescent patients. If a significant other has positive expectations, the trauma patient is often more likely to comply. On the other hand, respecting the patient's desire to keep communications confidential can also be key to developing an alliance. Large audiences of staff should be avoided.

> A 19-year-old female who was raped on a date after becoming intoxicated presents with agitation and threatened suicide:
>
> > **Patient:** I don't want my parents to know, but it is okay to talk with my sister.
> > **Staff:** Are you comfortable talking to us about this?
> > **Patient:** Yes. But I feel nervous in front of so many people.

Although the issue of retelling remains controversial, the value of crisis management is clearer. Assess real psychosocial needs. Does the traumatized patient need (consequent to the trauma) housing, clothes, money, support, sleep, food, contact with family, a letter to an employer, permission to take off time from work, and so forth? Often attempts at crisis management precede therapy work and strengthen the alliance.

The consequences for the patient of avoidant behavior—for example, not going to work or school, excessive sleeping—must be clearly assessed, understood, and addressed. Medication can be useful during this problem-solving effort.

Avoidance lends itself to behavioral, cognitive, and dynamic interventions. Not infrequently, multimodal approaches are used.

> **Staff:** So how have you been doing since this happened to you? [assessment]
> **Patient:** I can't study. I can't go to school after this happened.
> **Staff:** Is this an area in which you would like to have help? [alliance building]
> **Patient:** Definitely.

Some sample (simplified) problem-solving responses are

- *Behavioral:* Would it help if you cut back on the number of classes you were attending?
- *Cognitive:* What is your best/easiest subject? Do you think you can still do that?
- *Dynamic:* What feelings about what happened are making it hard to go back to school now?

Advocacy and education are frequently required in a trauma situation:

> **Mother:** When will she snap out of it?
> **Staff:** Your daughter plans to cut back on classes for a while; she is going to try very hard and will take one history class for now. She is concerned about you understanding how hard she is trying.

Regardless of one's theoretical approach, emphasis is placed on how the patient copes with trauma. One should always build on patients' strengths and coping mechanisms.

A 32-year-old emergency worker with no past psychiatric history has begun to ruminate about being alive after the collapse of a building that was attacked. He describes how the building collapsed and witnessing the loss of all the men in his command as well as that of people jumping out of the window.

Staff: What happened then?
Patient: I was lying there covered with debris. I could not feel my arm *(his arm was broken)*. I just wanted to lie there.
Staff: How did you get out?
Patient: I saw a lighted area after the dust cleared.
Staff: And then what did you do?
Patient: Then I thought of my three children. I wanted to see them. So I crawled out.
Staff: Have you seen them?
Patient *(with tears):* Yes!
Staff: You made the right choice.
Patient: I guess so.

Mardi Horowitz (1991) has developed a short-term dynamic therapy of stress response syndromes that emphasizes dealing with the intrusive and repetitive thoughts, denial, and numbing that often follow a traumatic experience. Horowitz attempts to examine the "person schema" and the need to change this schema. In essence, this "schema" is how a person consciously and, to some extent, unconsciously defines herself or himself. There is an emphasis on helping the patient control intrusive and often denigrating thoughts about the self.

The need for maintaining an optimal level of anxiety (usually lower than in outpatient work) and attending to agitation and psychotic features has already been emphasized. Patients in a crisis following trauma will often feel an urge to tell and retell in detail their painful experiences. Others will seal it over. Horowitz defines "dosing" as the regulation of the amount of material and distress the patient manifests during retelling.

In addition, coping mechanisms and styles will dictate the optimal limit-setting and focusing techniques. He distinguishes between a "hysterical style" and an "obsessional style." With the hysterical style, one needs to pursue details, encourage labeling of experience, and help the patient maintain focus. With an obsessional style, the staff needs to ask for overall impressions when the patient gets bogged down in details, help connect the patients to his or her emotions, focus on the actual images of events and their meanings rather than the words used to describe events, and watch for the shifting of meaning and tendency to procrastinate.

Conclusion

In this chapter, we have tried to review and illustrate psychological and psychosocial interventions that are inevitably involved in PES care. Despite the limitations of the time and milieu, productive work can be accomplished. Many process-oriented approaches can be added to assessment procedures, constituting a set of psychotherapy tools that decreases agitation and assaultiveness, indirectly increases efficiency, and improves long-term outcome. Diversity of experience and sharing among staff help to increase the repertoire of skills. The impulse to help others, when tempered with flexibility and pragmatism, makes this endeavor more meaningful and effective.

References

Adler G: Borderline personality disorders in the emergency room: current perspectives. Emergency Psychiatry 6(4):119–122, 2000

Allen MH, Currier GW, Hughes DH, et al: Treatment of Behavioral Emergencies (Postgraduate Medicine Expert Consensus Guideline Series). New York, McGraw-Hill, 2001

American Psychiatric Association: Practice guideline for the treatment of patients with borderline personality disorder. Am J Psychiatry 158(10, suppl):1–52, 2001

Beauford JE, McNiel DE, Binder RL: Utility of the initial therapeutic alliance in evaluating psychiatric patients' risk of violence. Am J Psychiatry 154(9):1272–1276, 1997

Beck AT: Cognitive Therapy and Emotional Disorders. New York, Internatinal Universities Press, 1976

Beck AT, Greenberg RL: Brief cognitive therapies. Psychiatr Clin North Am 2:23–37, 1979

Bergman MS, Hartman FR: The Evolution of Psychoanalytic Technique. New York, Basic Books, 1976

Berlin J: Psychological and psychodynamic approaches in the PES. Emergency Psychiatry 6:108–110, 2000

Bibring E: Contributions to the Symposium on the Theory of the Therapeutic Results of Psychoanalysis. Int J Psychoanal 18:170, 1937

Black KJ, Wilson M, Wetzel M: Assaults by patients on psychiatric residents at three training sites. Hosp Community Psychiatry 45:706–710, 1994

Bowen M: Family Therapy in Clinical Practice. New York, Jason Aronson, 1978

Caplan G: Principles of Preventative Psychotherapy. New York, Basic Books, 1964

Clarkin JF, Hurt SW, Crilly JL: Therapeutic alliance and hospital treatment outcome. Hosp Community Psychiatry 38:871–875, 1987

Copersino ML, Serper MR, Allen MH: Rapid screening for cognitive disorders. Emergency Psychiatry 4(3):51–53, 1998

Crits-Christoph P, Barber JP (eds): Handbook of Short-Term Dynamic Psychotherapy. New York, Basic Books, 1991

Davanloo H: Techniques of short-term dynamic psychotherapy. Psychiatr Clin North Am 2:11–22, 1979

Davanloo H: Short-Term Dynamic Psychotherapy. New York, Jason Aronson, 1980

Ellis A: Humanistic Psychotherapy: A Rational-Emotive Approach. New York, McGraw-Hill, 1973

Forster P: Accurate assessment of short-term suicide risk in a crisis. Psychiatric Annals 24(11):571–577, 1994

Gabbard GO: Psychodynamic Psychiatry in Clinical Practice, 3rd Edition. Washington, DC, American Psychiatric Press, 2000

Gerson B: Psychiatric emergencies and overview. Am J Psychiatry 137:1–9, 1980

Haley J: Problem-Solving Therapy, San Francisco, CA, Jossey-Bass, 1977

Horowitz MJ: Short-term dynamic therapy of stress response syndromes, in Handbook of Short-Term Dynamic Psychotherapy. Edited by Crits-Christoph P, Barber JP. New York, Basic Books, 1991, pp 166–198

Kane JM, Quitkin F, Rifkin A, et al: Attitudinal changes of involuntary patients following treatment. Arch Gen Psychiatry 40:374–377, 1983

Kass F, Karasu BT: Emergency room patients in concurrent therapy, a neglected clinical phenomenon. Am J Psychiatry 136:91–92, 1979

Kirtland CP, Prout MF, Schwarz RA: Posttraumatic Stress Disorder: A Clinician's Guide. New York, Plenum, 1991

Langs R: Unconscious communication in the emergency room. Emergency Psychiatry 6:111–112, 2000

Luborsky L: How to Maximize the Curative Factors in Dynamic Psychotherapy in Psychodynamic Treatment Research. New York, Basic Books, 1993, pp 519–535

Luborsky L, David M: Short-term supportive expressive psychoanalytic psychotherapy, in Handbook of Short-Term Dynamic Psychotherapy. Edited by Crits-Christoph P, Barber JP. New York, Basic Books, 1991, pp 110–132

Luborsky L, Crits-Christophe P, Alexander L, et al: Two helping alliance methods for predicting outcome of psychotherapy. J Nerv Ment Dis 171:480–489, 1983

Malan DH: The Frontier of Brief Psychotherapy. New York, Plenum, 1976

Mann J, Goldman J: A Casebook in Time-Limited Psychotherapy. New York, McGraw-Hill, 1982

Marmor J: Historical aspects of short-term dynamic psychotherapy. Psychiatr Clin North Am 2:3–9, 1979

Marziali E, Marmar C, Krupnick J: Therapeutic alliance scales: development and relationship to psychotherapy outcome. Am J Psychiatry 138:361–364, 1981

Meichenbaum D: Cognitive modification of test anxious college strudents. J Consult Clin Psychol 39:370–380, 1972

Meichenbaum M: Cognitive Behavioral Modification: An Integrative Approach. New York, Plenum, 1977

Melancon G, Boyer R: How to prevent post-traumatic stress disorder before traumatization occurs? Can J Psychiatry 44(3):253–258, 1999

Meyerson AT, Delaney B, Herbert J, et al: Do aspects of standard emergency care have potentially traumatic sequuelae? Emergency Psychiatry 4(3):44–48, 1998

Rabkin R: Strategic Psychotherapy: Brief and Symptomatic Treatment. New York, Basic Books, 1977

Rogers C: Client-Centered Therapy. Boston, MA, Houghton Mifflin, 1951

Rogers C: On Becoming a Person. Boston, MA, Houghton Mifflin, 1961

Rosenberg R: Psychological treatments in the psychiatric emergency sevice, in The Growth and Specialization of Emergency Psychiatry (New Directions for Mental Health Services, No 67). Edited by Allen MH. San Francisco, CA, Jossey-Bass, 1995, pp 77–85

Rosenberg R, Kesselman M: The therapeutic alliance and the psychiatric emergency room. Hosp Community Psychiatry 44:78–80, 1993

Satir V: Conjoint Family Therapy. Palo Alto, CA, Science & Behavior Books, 1983

Sifneos PE: Short-Term Dynamic Psychotherapy: Evaluation and Technique. New York, Plenum, 1979

Talmon M: Single-Session Therapy. San Francisco, CA, Jossey-Bass, 1990

Thienhaus OJ: Academic issues in emergency psychiatry, in The Growth and Specialization of Emergency Psychiatry (New Directions for Mental Health Services, No 67). Edited by Allen MH. San Francisco, CA, Jossey-Bass, 1995, pp 109–114

Van Gent EM, Zwart FM: Psychoeducation of partners of bipolar manic patients. J Affect Disord 21:15–18, 1991

Wallace BC: Treating crack cocaine dependence: the critical role of relapse prevention. J Psychoactive Drugs 24:213–222, 1992

Wessely S, Rose S, Bisson J: Brief psychological interventions (debriefing) for trauma-related symptoms and the prevention of posttraumatic stress disorder. Cochrane Database System Review 2000

Whitaker CA, Malone TP: The Roots of Psychotherapy. New York, Brunner/Mazel, 1981

Wolpe J: The Practice of Behavior Therapy, 4th Edition. Elmsford, NY, Pergamon, 1990

Zetzel E: The concept of transference. Int J Psychoanal 37:369–376, 1956

Additional Readings

American Psychiatric Association: Diagnostic and Statistical Manual of Mental Disorders, 4th Edition, Text Revision. Washington, DC, American Psychiaric Association, 2000

Beutler LE, Anderson L: Characteristics of the therapist in brief psychotherapy. Psychiatr Clin North Am 2(1):125–137, 1979

Brasch JS, Davies G: Teaching trainees to assess agitated patients. Emergency Psychiatry 7(2):41–42,

Bremner JD:Alterations in brain structure and function associated with post-traumatic stress disorder. Semin Clin Neuropsychiatry 4(4): 249–255, 1999

Chambers RA, Bremner JD, Moghaddam B, et al: Glutamate and post-traumatic stress disorder: toward a psychobiology of dissociation. Semin Clin Neuropsychiatry 4(4):274–281, 1999

Connor KM, Davidson JR, Weisler RH, et al: A pilot study of mirtaza-pine in post-traumatic stress disorder. Int Clin Psychopharmacol 14(1):29–31, 1999a

Connor KM, Sutherland SM, Tupler LA: Fluoxetine in post-traumatic stress disorder: randomised, double-blind study. Br J Psychiatry 175:17–22, 1999b

Corey G: Theory and Practice of Counseling and Psychotherapy, 5th Edition. Pacific Grove, CA, Brooks/Cole, 1996

Cusack K, Spates CR: EMDR treatment of posttraumatic stress disorder (PTSD). J Anxiety Disord 13(1–2):87–99, 1999

Dalery J, Rochet T: Acute exacerbations in schizophrenia. Encephale 25 (spec no 3):5–8 , 1999

Forster P, King JK: Definitive treatments of patients with serious mental disorders in an emergency service. Hosp Community Psychiatry 45: 867–869, 1117–1118, 1994

Freedman SA, Brandes D, Peri T, et al: Predictors of chronic post-trau-matic stress disorder: a prospective study. Br J Psychiatry 174:353–359, 1999

Guderman JE: Psychodynamic approaches to the person with psychosis in the emergency situation. Emergency Psychiatry 6:113–116, 2000

Krashin D, Oates EW: Risperidone as an adjunct therapy for post-trau-matic stress disorder. Mil Med 164(8):605–606, 1999

Maes M, Lin AH, Verkerk R, et al: Serotonergic and noradrenergic markers of post-traumatic stress disorder with and without major depression. Neuropsychopharmacology 20(2):188–197, 1999

Miller NE, Luborsky L, Barber JP, et al: Psychodynamic Treatment Research: A Handbook for Clinical Practice. New York, Basic Books, 1993

Ohry A, Rattok J, Solomon Z: Post-traumatic stress disorder in brain injury patients. Brain Inj 10(9):687–695, 1996

Peterson KC, Prout MF, Schwarz RA: Post-Traumatic Stress Disorder: A Clinician's Guide. New York, Plenum, 1990

Piper WE: Psychotherapy research in the 1980s: defining areas of con-sensus and controversy. Hosp Community Psychiatry 39:1055–1064, 1988

Roberts AR: Crisis Intervention Handbook: Assessment, Treatment, and Research. Belmont, CA, Wadsworth, 1990

Rosenfarb IS, Neuchterlein KH, Goldstein MJ, et al: Neurocognitive vulnerability, interpersonal criticism, and the emergence of unusual thinking by schizophrenic patients during family transactions. Arch Gen Psychiatry 57:1174–1179, 2000

Schuster JM: Frustration or opportunity? The impact of managed care on emergency psychiatry, in The Growth and Specialization of Emergency Psychiatry (New Directions for Mental Health Services, No 67). Edited by Allen MH. San Francisco, CA, Jossey-Bass, 1995, pp 101–108

Skodol AE: Problems in Differential Diagnosis: From DSM-III to DSM-III-R in Clinical Practice. Washington, DC, American Psychiatric Press, 1989

Stein MB, Koverola C, Hanna C, et al: Hippocampal volume in women victimized by childhood sexual abuse. Psychol Med 27(4):951–959, 1997

Whitehorn JC, Betz B: A study of psychotherapeutic relationships between physicians and schizophrenic patients. Am J Psychiatry 111: 321–331, 1954

Zimmerman M, Mattia JI: Psychotic subtyping of major depressive disorder and posttraumatic stress disorder. J Clin Psychiatry 60(5):311–314, 1999

Index

*Page numbers printed in **boldface** type refer to tables.*

Biological factors, and
aggression, 122–123
Bipolar disorder
aggression, 126
suicide and suicidal ideation,
78, 87, 88, 102, 103
Borderline personality disorder
psychosocial interventions,
167
suicide and suicide attempts,
78, 89
Brief therapy
dynamic approaches to
psychosocial intervention,
167–168
suicidal patients, 100

California, psychiatric
emergency services and
involuntary admissions, 51,
52
California Verbal Learning Test
(CVLT), 64–66
Cancer, and suicide, 90, 91
Cardiovascular disorders, and
psychiatric symptoms, 40
Carve-outs, and managed care,
19
CASE (Chronological
Assessment of Suicide
Events), 93–94
Case management
managed care, 19–20, 22
mobile team model, 17
Catastrophizing, and automatic
thinking, 163
Centers for Medicare and
Medicaid Services (CMS),
Hospital Conditions of
Participation for Patients'
Rights, 136

Central nervous system (CNS)
infection, 39
Cerebral atrophy, 38
Checklist, for triage, 56, 57. *See
also* Guidelines
Chest, inspection and
auscultation of, 46
Chloral hydrate, 142
Chlorpromazine, 140
Chronic obstructive pulmonary
disease (COPD), 39
Clock Drawing Test (CDT), 66–67
Clonazepam
agitation and aggression, 138
suicidal patients, 102
Clozapine, 103
Cognitive therapy, and
psychosocial interventions,
162–165. *See also* Cognitive-
behavioral therapy
Cognitive-behavioral
modification (CBM), 164
Cognitive-behavioral therapy, for
suicidal patients, 100. *See also*
Behavioral therapy;
Cognitive therapy
Cognitive impairment
agitation, 118
automatic thinking, 163–164
medical assessment, 45
psychiatric assessment and
screening procedures,
62–67
Collateral contact, 94
Communication
consultation model, 7
family therapy, 173
paranoid patients, 134
specialized psychiatric
emergency services
model, 10

Community service providers,
and crisis hospitalization, 13
Compliance
as risk factor for violence, 129
treatment for suicidal patients,
95
Computed tomography (CT)
scans, 43
Computerized records, and
future of psychiatric
emergency services, 26–28
Conduct disorder, 129
Confidentiality
computerized records, 28
suicidal patients, 94
Congestive heart failure, 39
Consortium model, 25
Consultation model, for
psychiatric services in
emergency departments,
3–4, 6–8
Contact time, and managed care,
20–21
Continuity of care
as goal of psychiatric
emergency services, 6
as risk factor for suicide, 86–87
Coping strategies, and
psychosocial interventions
for trauma, 175, 176, 177
Cost
effectiveness of mobile team
model, 15
medical assessment, 46
Countertransference, and
suicidal patients, 93, 97, 98
County drift, and access to
psychiatric services, 5
Crisis hospitalization model,
11–14. *See also*
Hospitalization

Crisis intervention
psychosocial interventions,
157–158
suicidal patients, 100
Crisis management, and
psychosocial interventions
for trauma, 176
Crisis residences model, 17–18
Crisis Triage Rating Scale (CTRS),
56–58
Cultural issues, and family
therapy, 173

Dangerousness, and involuntary
civil commitment, 52. *See also*
Violence and violent
behavior
Day hospital programs, and
managed care, 21
Debriefing
psychosocial interventions
and therapeutic alliance,
156
treatment of agitation or
aggression, 132
Defenses, and dynamic
psychotherapy, 169
Delirium, and agitation, 120
Delusional disorder, 117
Dementia
agitation and aggression, 118,
120, 126
cognitive screening, 62, 65, 66,
67
Depression
agitation, 119–120
hospitalization, 53
as risk factor for suicide, 87, 88,
89, 90, 101, 125
Desensitization, 162
Desipramine, 101

Diabetes, 40

Diagnosis. *See also* Assessment
    agitation and aggression,
        116–118
    psychiatric assessment and
        definitive, 50, 53–55, 61

Diphenhydramine, 142

Disposition, and psychiatric
    assessment, 50–52, 60

Distance decay phenomenon, 5

Divalproex sodium, 14

Documentation, or seclusion and
    restraint episodes, 137

Dopamine antagonists, and
    agitation, 120

Dosages, of medications for
    aggression and agitation,
    140, 141

Droperidol, 140

Dynamic approaches, to
    psychosocial intervention,
    165–170

Education, and psychosocial
    interventions for trauma, 176

Elderly. *See also* Age
    dosages of antipsychotics, 141
    medical assessment and
        changes in mental status,
        44, 48

Electrocardiographic screening,
    and medical assessment, 43

Electroconvulsive therapy (ECT),
    and suicidal patients, 101

Electoencephalograms, and
    violent behavior, 123–124

Electrolyte imbalances, 39

Emergency, definition of, 1, 58

Emergency departments (EDs)
    access to health care, 3
    agitation and aggression, 131

consultation model, 6
delivery of psychiatric
    services, 3
risk assessment for suicide,
    91–94

Emergency Medical Treatment
    and Active Labor Act
    (EMTALA), 3, 58–59

Emotions, and therapeutic
    alliance, 156–157

Empathy, and therapeutic
    alliance, 156

Empowerment, and person-
    centered therapy, 171

Endocrine disorders, and
    psychiatric symptoms, 40

Environmental risk factors, for
    violence, 129–130

Epidemiology, of suicide, 75–76

Epilepsy, 40. *See also* Seizures;
    Temporal lobe epilepsy

Equilibrium, and crisis
    intervention, 158

Ethics, and treatment for suicidal
    patients, 99

Ethnicity, and risk factors for
    suicide, 82

Excess mortality, in emergency
    care patients, 91–92

Exploratory-supportive
    intervention continuum,
    165–167

Extrapyramidal side effects
    (EPS), and antipsychotics,
    139–140, 141

Family, and specialized
    psychiatric emergency
    services model, 9. *See also*
    Family therapy

Family-based crisis home, 18

Human immunodeficiency virus
(HIV), prevalence of in
psychiatric patients, 37.
See also AIDS
Huntington's disease, 65
Hypertensive encephalopathy, 39
Hypothalamic-pituitary-adrenal
(HPA) axis, and agitation, 119
Hysterical style, and coping
mechanisms, 177–178

Impulsive violence, 116
Impulsivity
involuntary civil commitment,
52
suicide attempts, 78
Informed consent, and research
in psychiatric emergency
services, 24
Insomnia, and anxiety, 97
Integrated psychiatric emergency
service, 4
Intelligence (IQ) scores, and
violence, 124
Intensive Short-term Dynamic
Psychotherapy, 168–169
Interrater reliability, of psychiatric assessment, 54–55
Interviews
behavioral therapy for
agitation and aggression,
132
psychosocial interventions
and therapeutic alliance,
155–157
risk assessment for violent
behavior, 130
Intracranial aneurysm, 39
Intramuscular administration, of
medications for agitation and
aggression, 138, 140, 141

Involuntary civil commitment,
and psychiatric assessment,
50, 51–53
Involuntary medication
administration, 138, 139
Irritability
mania, 118
psychosocial interventions
and therapeutic alliance,
157

Joint Commission on Accreditation of Healthcare Organizations (JCAHO), 135, 136

Labeling and mislabeling, and
automatic thinking, 163
Laboratory tests, and medical
assessment, 42, 46
Leader, and family network, 172
Legal issues
managed care, 22
suicide and suicidal ideation,
104–105
triage, 58–59
Life satisfaction, and risk factors
for suicide, 85–86
Lithium, and suicidal patients,
102–103
Long-term treatment, for suicidal
patients, 101–104
Lorazepam, and agitation or
aggression, 138, 140, 141
Lumbar puncture tests, 43
Lupus, 39

Magnification, and automatic
thinking, 163
Malpractice liability, and
treatment of suicidal
patients, 96, 104–105

Normal-pressure hydrocephalus, 39

Nurses. *See also* Staff and staffing
  psychiatric assessment, 61
  triage, 55–56

Nutritional deficiencies, and psychiatric symptoms, 40

Observation, and crisis hospitalization model, 12

Obsessional style, and coping mechanisms, 177–178

Ocular examination, 45

Olanzapine, 103, 141

Oral administration, of medications for agitation and aggression, 138

Organic brain syndromes. *See also* Medical conditions
  deficiencies in medical assessment, 48
  exacerbation of mental illness, 40

Outreach, and mobile team model, 15–16, 17

Overgeneralization, and automatic thinking, 163

Overt Aggression Scale, 142

Panic disorder, and agitation, 120

Paranoia, and communication, 134

Paranoid schizophrenia, 117

Pathophysiology
  of aggression, 122–126
  of agitation, 119–122

Performance-based cognitive screening examinations, 63

Person-centered therapy, and psychosocial interventions, 170–172

Personality disorders
  aggression, 125
  crisis hospitalization model, 13
  risk factors for suicide, 87, 89, 90

Personalization, and automatic thinking, 163

Personnel qualifications, and assessment, 49–50, 61

Pharmacotherapy, for agitation and aggression, 137–142. *See also* Antidepressants; Antipsychotics; Medication

Physical examinations, 41–42, 47

Physical plant, and consultation model, 7

Physical restraints, and treatment of agitation and aggression, 135–137

Physicians. *See also* Staff and staffing
  consultation model, 7
  failure to document suicide history, 76
  orders for seclusion or restraints, 136

Planning, of treatment for suicidal patients, 103–104

Pneumonia, 39

Polarized thinking, 163

Police, and mobile team model, 16

Positron emission tomography (PET), and violent behavior, 123–124

Posttraumatic stress disorder (PTSD)
  psychosocial interventions, 174–178
  as risk factor for suicide, 89

Power, and person-centered
therapy, 172
Precertification, managed care, 21
Prediction, of suicide, 79–80
Premeditated violence, 116
Prevalence
of medical morbidity in
psychiatric patients, 37, 38
of missed physical diagnoses,
47–48
of suicide and suicide
attempts, 76, 87, 90
Prevention
of posttraumatic stress
disorder, 174–175
of suicide, 95–96
Preventive medical care, and
psychiatrists, 50
Problem-solving, and
psychosocial interventions
for trauma, 176
Procedural approach, to psychosocial intervention, 153
Process approach, to
psychosocial intervention,
153
Protective factors, and suicide, 91
Psychiatric disorders
aggressive behavior, 117
as risk factors for suicide, 83,
87–90
Psychiatric emergency services
(PESs). See also Aggression;
Agitation; Assessment;
Psychosocial interventions;
Suicide and suicidal ideation
as care setting for psychotherapy, 151
definition of, 1
future directions of, 25–28
goals for, 4–6

managed care, 18–22
medical emergencies and
psychiatry, 2–4
models for delivery of services,
6–18
research in, 23–25
teaching as role of, 22–23
Psychiatric house calls, and
mobile team model, 16
Psychiatrists. See also Staff and
staffing
consultation model, 8
medical assessment and
training of, 36–37, 49–50
specialized psychiatric
emergency services
model, 10
Psychodynamic therapy, 167
Psychoeducation, and family
therapy, 173–174
Psychosis and psychotic
disorders
agitation, 120–122
assessment, 5, 51
suicide and suicidal ideation,
89, 101
psychosocial interventions,
155, 162
violence and agitation, 117
Psychosocial assessment, 59–60,
152, 153. See also Assessment
Psychosocial interventions
crisis intervention, 157–158
goals of in emergencies, 152
linear versus flexible process,
152–154
suicide and suicidal ideation,
100
therapeutic alliance, 154–157
therapy work, 158–178
Pulmonary embolism, 39

Sexual orientation, and suicide in adolescents, 83–84
Short-term dynamic therapy, and stress response syndromes, 177
Short-Term Supportive Expressive Psychoanalytic Psychotherapy, 169–170
Social isolation, as risk factor for suicide, 90
Social workers, and psychiatric assessment, 49, 61
Socioeconomic status
    as risk factor for suicide, 84
    as risk factor for violence, 128
Sodium amobarbital, 142
Somatic conditions, and psychiatric symptoms, 40
Space
    organization of in emergency departments, 7
    specialized psychiatric emergency services model, 9–10
Specialized psychiatric emergency service model, 4, 8–11
Special populations
    medical assessment of psychiatric patients, 48
    psychosocial interventions, 167
Stabilization, as goal of psychiatric emergency services, 5
Staff and staffing. See also Nurses; Physicians; Psychiatrists
    emergency departments and attitudes toward psychiatric emergencies, 8
    physical restraints, 136–137

specialized psychiatric emergency services model, 9, 10
    timely rendering of psychiatric emergency care, 4
Subcortical dementia, 65, 67
Subdural hematoma, 39
Substance abuse
    assessment, 5
    cognitive deficits, 64–65
    crisis hospitalization model, 13
    psychiatric emergencies, 2
    psychiatric symptoms, 39
    suicide and suicidal ideation, 83, 89
    therapeutic alliance, 155
    toxicology screens, 42–43
    violence, 116
Substance-induced agitation, 120
Substance-induced mood disorder, 78
Suicide and suicidal ideation. See also Violence and violent behavior
    assessment, 5, 78–80
    crisis hospitalization model, 13
    epidemiology, 75–76
    guidelines for risk assessment, 59
    interventions and treatment, 94–104
    medical-legal issues, 104–105
    norepinephrine levels, 124
    psychiatric emergencies, 2
    risk factors, 81–91
    serotonergic system, 125
    spectrum of behavior, 77–78
Supervision, of suicidal patients, 95
Supportive interventions, 165–167

Sweden, antidepressants and suicide rates, 102
Syphilis, 39

Talking down, and agitation or aggression, 132
Teaching, as function of psychiatric emergency services, 22–23
Temporal arteritis, 39
Temporal lobe epilepsy, aggression, 118. *See also* Epilepsy
Temporal lobe lesions, and aggression, 123
Therapeutic alliance
    psychosocial interventions, 154–157, 172
    suicidal patients, 97
Therapy work, and psychosocial interventions, 158–178
Thought and thinking
    automatic thinking and psychosocial interventions, 163–164
    as risk factor for suicide, 77, 81–82
Three Ratings of Involuntary Admissibility (TRIAD), 51, 52
Thyroid disease, 39
Thyroid function tests, 43
Timely rendering, of psychiatric emergency care, 4
Time outs, and agitation or aggression, 132, 134–135
Toxicology screens, and substance abuse, 42–43
Trailmaking Test (TMT), 63–64
Transference
    dynamic psychotherapy, 169
    suicidal patients, 97
Transnosological syndromes, 115

Trauma, and psychosocial interventions, 174–178
Trazodone, 101
Treatment. *See also* Cognitive-behavioral therapy; Pharmacotherapy; Psychosocial interventions
    agitation and aggression, 130–142
    suicide and suicidal ideation, 79–80, 94–104
Triage
    medical assessment, 43–45
    psychiatric assessment, 55–59
    skills required, 151–152
    suicide attempts and ideation, 80
Triangles of person and of action, in dynamic psychotherapy, 168–169
Tricyclic antidepressants, and suicidal patients, 101. *See also* Antidepressants
Tumors, and psychiatric symptoms, 39

Unemployment, as risk factor for suicide, 84
Unipolar depression, 78
University of Cincinnati Hospital, 48–49
Urinary tract infection, 39

Valproate, and aggression, 126
Valproic acid, and agitation, 120
Vascular dementia, 67
Vasculitis, 39
Verbal techniques, for treatment of agitation and aggression, 133–134